Co-Occurring Disorders Recovery Workbook

by Dennis C. Daley, Ph.D.

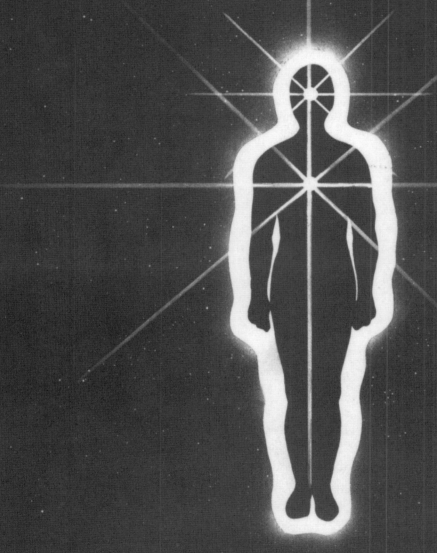

Strategies to Manage Substance Use and Mental Health Disorders

Foreword by Terence T. Gorski

© 2011

Dennis C. Daley, Ph.D.

Dual Disorders Recovery Counseling: Integrated Treatment for Substance Use and Mental Health Disorders is the companion clinician's manual that can be used with this client workbook. Both the client workbook and clinician manual are available from the publisher:

Herald Publishing House/Independence Press
1001 West Walnut Street
P.O. Box 390
Independence, MO 64051-0390
Phone: 1-800-767-8181 or (816) 521-3015

Author's Note:

Thanks to Cindy Hurney for helping to update this workbook. Her creativity and attention to detail are appreciated. Cindy has helped with all of my publications over the past two decades and her work is outstanding. I would also like to thank Gretchen Booz for her support and friendship over many years. Thanks also to Mary Kay Speaks for all the time and excellent work editing this version of the workbook. Last, thanks to my long-time colleague Terence Gorski for his support of my writings, and for his many contributions to the field of treatment and recovery from addiction and co-occurring disorders.

ISBN: 978-0-8309-1501-9

Table of Contents

Foreword by Terence T. Gorski

The treatment of clients with co-occurring or dual disorders (the combination of a substance use disorder and psychiatric illness) is a significant problem for professionals in addiction medicine and mental health treatment settings. Many studies show high rates of co-occurring disorders and that "integrated" treatment is the optimal approach to care and reduces the risk of relapse to either disorder.

I have known Dennis C. Daley for nearly 25 years and am impressed by the extensive work he has done in the field of co-occurring disorders. Dennis and his colleagues at the University of Pittsburgh Medical Center's Addiction Medicine Services (AMS) were one of the first groups of professionals in the United States to develop treatment programs for clients who have both substance use (addiction) and psychiatric disorders. Dennis has been "down in the trenches" working with clients for decades and understands the many challenges of recovery. In addition to his clinical work, Dennis has been involved in research for over two decades and has helped to advance our understanding of addiction and co-occurring disorders. He was the first in the United States to actually develop interactive recovery workbooks for clients with co-occurring disorders. His work and materials are used in many treatment programs in the United States and other countries.

This updated *Co-Occurring Disorders Recovery Workbook* presents many proven strategies that can help clients recover from their disorders. As I reviewed this guide, I was impressed with the clear, concise and understandable way in which Dennis presents material. This workbook can be used in individual and group counseling. Families can also benefit from information presented in it as well. Dennis remains a strong advocate for families and children and urges clients to evaluate the impact of their disorders on the family, including children.

Many readers are familiar with my work on relapse prevention and know that failure to address mental health problems while in recovery from an addiction raises the risk of relapse. Dennis includes considerable attention on the problem of relapse and provides strategies to reduce the risk of relapse, both to the addiction and the psychiatric illness.

I strongly believe that this *Co-Occurring Disorders Recovery Workbook* is one of the most comprehensive and important recovery guides in the field of treatment. Users of this guide who put forth time and effort in their recovery can benefit immensely from using the material presented.

Terence T. Gorski

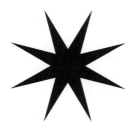

SECTION I

Understanding Co-Occurring Disorders and Recovery

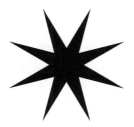

1. How to Use This Recovery Workbook

This recovery workbook was written for individuals recovering from both a substance use disorder (also called addiction or chemical dependency) and a psychiatric disorder (also called a mental health problem or mental disorder). It can help you regardless of the types and combinations of disorders you are recovering from. Having both a substance use and a psychiatric disorder is referred to as "co-occurring disorders."

You will learn about causes, effects and treatment of these disorders, strategies to aid recovery and reduce relapse risk, specific steps you can take to manage the challenges of recovery and how to take an active role in changing. You will also learn how mutual support programs like Alcoholics Anonymous (AA), Narcotics Anonymous (NA), Dual Recovery Anonymous (DRA), other Twelve-Step programs and others can help you.

This workbook has been used by tens of thousands of individuals for more than 20 years. The content reflects input from hundreds of patients in treatment who shared what they thought were important issues to discuss, information from research, professional writings and recovery literature, my decades of experiences as a therapist, teacher and researcher, and the experiences of numerous individuals in recovery. Topics of this recovery workbook include a range of issues relevant to all areas of recovery: physical, emotional or mental, social, family, spiritual and financial. Use any or all parts of this workbook to help you develop or improve coping skills to manage your disorders.

Specific topics in this workbook include:

- Understanding mental health (psychiatric illness) and addictive disorders

- Identifying why you came to treatment and setting goals

- Working through denial and overcoming roadblocks to recovery

- Understanding the recovery process from co-occurring disorders

- Motivating yourself to change and dealing with periods of low motivation

- Understanding the effects of co-occurring disorders on you and others

- Managing feelings such as anger, anxiety, boredom, and depression

- Changing behaviors

- Changing your thinking

- Developing your spirituality

- Developing structure and a daily plan of recovery

- Improving family and personal relationships

- Coping with social pressures to use alcohol or drugs or stop taking medications

- Building a support system or recovery network

- Making lifestyle changes

- Knowing the importance of follow-up treatment after participation in hospital based or residential treatment

- Using AA/NA/DRA, mental health support groups, and recovery clubs
- Developing a relapse prevention plan
- Having an emergency plan in case you feel suicidal, your psychiatric disorder worsens or you return to alcohol or drug use

Go at your own pace in recovery. Do not rush through this workbook. Take things slowly and focus on one or two changes at a time. Sometimes it helps to work on one section and "test out" new ideas before going on to the next section. You can use this workbook over a long period of time.

Be as honest as you can when working in this guide. Discuss your struggles or difficulties with your therapist or sponsor.

The sections you work on depend on your personal problems and needs as well as the length of time you are in treatment. Discuss completed sections with a member of your treatment team or sponsor. They can give you valuable feedback and guide you in selecting sections to work on.

This workbook was designed to help you develop your personal recovery plan. Be realistic when setting goals for change. Accept even small steps of change as a sign of improvement. Don't get down on yourself if you make a mistake or have a setback. Keep working your recovery plan and things will get better. It is your responsibility to read and finish assignments. It requires you to take an active role in your treatment. You have a big say in getting well and making positive changes. Change is hard, but you can do it. Keep trying. Keep all of your scheduled treatment appointments with your therapist or doctor. If you want to stop treatment, feel upset, angry or frustrated with your treatment, talk it over with your therapist. Together, you can figure out what's going on to make you feel this way.

Sharing your "story" and experiences with co-occurring disorders is an important part of recovery. Talking about your problems, symptoms, feelings, and completed assignments with your peers in group sessions, or with a counselor in individual sessions, allows you to get feedback from others.

As you recover from your disorders you will experience improvements in your health, which in turn, should lead to a better quality of life. Remember, no matter what disorders you have or how severe they are, you can get better. You can change. You can recover, but you need not do this alone.

Share Your Feedback about the Workbook

If you want to share your opinion about this workbook (what you liked and found helpful as well as ideas for improvement) send an e-mail to the author at *daleypublications@yahoo.com*. Your comments may help improve future editions of this workbook, which can benefit others in recovery.

Share Your Story of Recovery

You can also share your story with the author by sending it to the e-mail address above. It may be shared with others (first names only) on his webpage. If you share your story, be brief. Use a single paragraph to briefly summarize your substance use and mental health problem. You can share what type of substance use disorder you have, for how long, and how it has affected you and others. Do the same for your mental health disorder. Most of what you share should be your experiences of positive change—what you did in treatment and recovery to manage your disorders and improve yourself and the quality of your life. Others will benefit more from hearing about what you did to help yourself and make positive changes than they will hearing the details of your disorders. If the author shares any of your personal story on his webpage to help others, your name will not be used to maintain confidentiality.

2. *Understanding Mental Health and Substance Use Disorders*

The National Institute of Mental Health conducted a major study of adults in the United States to determine how many had a mental health or alcohol and drug problem at some point in their lives.[1] The results of this study showed over 22 percent of adults, either currently or in the past, have had a mental health problem; 29 percent of these also had an alcohol or drug problem at some time in their lives. This study also showed that over 16 percent of adults, either currently or in the past, have had an alcohol or drug problem; 37 percent of those with an alcohol problem and 53 percent of those with a drug problem also had a mental health problem at some time in their lives.

Another large scale study called the National Comorbidity Study (NCS) also found high rates of co-occurring disorders.[2] The NCS study found that 51 percent of people with a psychiatric disorder had an alcohol or drug problem at some point in their lives, and 41–66 percent of people with an alcohol or drug problem had a psychiatric disorder at some point in their lives.

Many other studies of people seeking care for psychiatric illness or an alcohol or drug problem also show that many people have more than one disorder.[3, 4] Some people have two or more different psychiatric disorders in addition to an alcohol or drug problem. One of the studies that I conducted found an average of 3.13 diagnoses among dual diagnosis patients.[5]

Since alcohol and drug problems affect mental health disorders and recovery, and since mental health disorders affect the use of alcohol or other drugs or recovery, treatment must address both disorders together. Focusing on recovery from only one of your disorders puts you at risk to relapse to the other. "Integrated" treatment gives you the best chance of recovery.

Substance Use Disorders

Many different legal and illegal substances are used and abused by people with psychiatric disorders. These include nicotine, alcohol, marijuana, crack or cocaine, other stimulants, opiates such as heroin or prescription pain medications, tranquilizers (also called sedatives), PCP, hallucinogens, and inhalants. The number one drug of abuse remains alcohol. In fact, many more people die each year or experience serious medical or life problems from alcohol than cocaine or other street drugs. While street drugs such as crack cocaine, heroin, or marijuana are abused by many people with psychiatric disorders, so are prescribed drugs such as tranquilizers or pain medications. Many people get hooked on prescription drugs initially taken for medical or psychiatric symptoms. Some of these people exhibit "drug seeking" behaviors. They go from doctor to doctor or make multiple visits to emergency rooms or urgent care clinics to get drugs for a variety of complaints or symptoms such as anxiety, sleep difficulties or pain. As soon as they think a particular drug isn't helpful, they increase the amount without medical supervision or talking with their therapist or doctor. Or, they seek other types of medications. The result is that they become addicted to prescription drugs, which can interfere with recovery from other addictions and their psychiatric illness.

Substance use disorders (SUDs) refer to any type of problem with alcohol or drugs. These problems vary from mild to severe and life threatening. The more severe type of SUD is addiction (also called dependence). Similar to other diseases or illnesses, addiction has a cluster of symptoms. According to the American Psychiatric Association, you meet the criteria for addiction (dependence) if you show a problematic pattern of substance use causing problems in your life or personal distress. You have an addiction if you have shown three or more of the following symptoms related to your alcohol or drug use during the past 12 months: [6]

- Change in tolerance (significant increase or decrease).

- Withdrawal symptoms when you cut down or stop using substances.

- Using alcohol or drugs to avoid withdrawal symptoms.

- Having trouble cutting down or stopping once you drink or take drugs.

- Quitting for a period of time only to go back to using again.

- Spending a good deal of time to get, use or recover from effects of substances.

- Giving up important activities due to your alcohol or drug use.

- Continuing to use substances even though such use causes you problems.

If you have less than three of these symptoms and your life is harmed in some way as a result of your use, your condition is referred to as substance abuse.[7] A big mistake many people make is believing that they have to be "physically addicted" to alcohol or drugs or use almost every day in order to qualify for having an addiction. Nothing could be further from the truth. Many people who don't use every day and who don't show every symptom listed above still have a serious problem with alcohol or other drugs. Therefore, keep in mind that either "substance abuse or dependence" can cause much heartache and suffering, and interfere with recovery from psychiatric illness.

Even if you do not meet criteria for "abuse or dependence" your use of alcohol or other drugs can cause problems or intervention with your recovery from a psychiatric illness. Small amounts of drugs or alcohol can have more of a negative effect on a person with certain types of psychiatric illness such as psychotic or borderline disorders. For example, smoking pot may have mild effects on a person without a psychiatric illness. A person with schizophrenia may become more paranoid or psychotic after smoking marijuana.

Chapters 5 and 6 of this guide will help you examine your history of alcohol and other drug use, and the effects on your life. Completing the tasks in these chapters will help you determine the severity of your substance use and mental health related problems.

Acute and Chronic or Persistent Psychiatric Illness

Some people have only one or two *acute* episodes of a psychiatric illness during their lifetime. They do not experience their illness throughout their lives. Other people have *recurrent* psychiatric illness and experience three or more episodes throughout their lives. There may be years between episodes of illness. Many others experience some symptoms continuously over time. This is called *chronic or persistent* psychiatric illness. This type of illness is usually more disabling and often requires long-term care under the direction of a psychiatrist, psychologist, or other mental health professional. However, many people with chronic psychiatric illness have periods in which they do well and their symptoms remain controlled.

Types of Psychiatric Disorders

There are many different types of illnesses among adults. They show in symptoms related to your moods, thoughts, behaviors, and ability to function in your daily life. Keep in mind that you may have some symptoms from many disorders, but this does not mean you have a disorder. A disorder is diagnosed only when a pattern of symptoms has been present for a period of time and causes personal distress and/or problems in your life. The most common categories of psychiatric illness found among people who have drug or alcohol use disorders include the following:

Mood Disorders

These include disturbances in your mood or how you feel.[8–11] The most common is *major depression* which involves feeling sad or blue, loss or decreased interest in life, difficulty concentrating, appetite or sleep problems, decline in energy, feelings of guilt and worthlessness and suicidal thoughts or actions. These symptoms are present most of the time, nearly every day for two weeks or longer.

Another type of mood disorder is called *recurrent depression*. This condition refers to having three or more different episodes of depression over time. Months or years may separate the episodes of depression. *Seasonal depression* refers to episodes of depression that tend to occur during specific times of the year such as during the winter. *Dysthymia* refers to a more chronic type of depression in which symptoms are more or less experienced for a long time, often two years or longer.

In some cases of depression, suicide is planned or even attempted. Drinking alcohol or taking other drugs can raise the risk of suicide because substances either impair judgment or give the person courage to try suicide.[12]

Some people switch back and forth between depression and mania, while others experience just one of these mood disorders. People who have both types of mood disorders have *"bipolar disorder"* or *"manic-depressive illness."* Some even experience symptoms of both depression and mania at the same time, a condition referred to as *"bipolar disorder, mixed."*

Mania is the opposite of depression in that the mood is very "high" instead of low.[13, 14] Energy and activity levels increase and the need for sleep decreases. The person is easily distracted and their thoughts may race. During a conversation, they may jump from topic to topic. Since their judgment is affected, they may do foolish things, go on spending sprees, put themselves in danger, or get involved in a lot of activities at once.

Some people experience symptoms of mania but do not have enough symptoms to meet criteria for bipolar illness. Plus, the symptoms may not cause severe problems often associated with bipolar illness. This form of mood disorder is called *cyclothymia*.

Drugs and alcohol are often abused during the time in which the person's mood is elevated. Patients sometimes talk about missing the "high mood" associated with bipolar disorder and may use cocaine or other stimulant drugs to recapture that "high" feeling.

Anxiety Disorders

These involve worrying too much, feeling a sense of dread or feeling very anxious.[15, 16] These usually include both physical and mental symptoms that affect the person's life and ability to function. Symptoms of anxiety may also be present in other psychiatric disorders such as depression. Many people get hooked on alcohol or drugs like tranquilizers as a way of reducing their anxiety symptoms. In the long-run however, things get worse because an addiction develops.

A *phobia* is an irrational fear of a situation or object so strong that it causes distress and problems in the person's life.[17] *Social phobias* involve irrational and intense fears of being looked at, criticized or rejected by others, or acting in ways that will be embarrassing or humiliating. Some people have many social situations they are afraid of while others have only one or two situations they fear. Social phobias include dating, speaking, writing or eating in public, or taking tests. *Simple phobias* involve irrational fears of situations such as being in a closed space, being in a high place, traveling by bus or plane, or fears of objects such as bugs, snakes, blood, or needles. One type of phobia, called *agoraphobia*, often makes the person a prisoner at home due to the fear of leaving. The person may never or seldom leave home as a result. A phobia usually is not based on reality and causes the person to avoid the situation or object that is feared.

Panic disorder involves sudden attacks in which the person feels an intense and overwhelming feeling of terror.[18] The person may worry about going crazy, dying, or feel that things "don't seem real." The person may feel dizzy or faint, shake or tremble, sweat, feel sick to the stomach, experience hot or cold flashes, or even feel chest pains or a racing heart.

Obsessive-compulsive disorder involves repeating behaviors like hand washing; checking doors, windows, or the stove; or counting objects many times.[19] The person often believes bad things will happen if these rituals are not repeated a certain number of times. This disorder also involves the recurrence of obsessions or senseless and frightening thoughts, over and over again.

Generalized anxiety disorder involves more or less continuous, unrealistic and excessive anxiety and worry about two or more areas of life.[20] This anxiety and worry is accompanied by other symptoms such as trembling, feeling shaky, feeling restless, shortness of breath, increased heart rate, feeling dizzy, nausea, hot flashes or chills, feeling hyper, keyed up or on edge, trouble concentrating or "going blank," and irritability.

Post-traumatic stress disorder (PTSD) may follow a psychologically upsetting event such as combat, torture, a serious threat to one's life or that of family or close friends, rape, or destruction of one's home or community as a result of a disaster.[21, 22] This event comes back in the form of recurrent dreams or thoughts about it or feeling like it is happening again. Seeing things that are a reminder of the event can cause severe distress. People with PTSD avoid things associated with the trauma or feel "numb" about it and detach from others as a result. Other symptoms of PTSD include trouble sleeping or concentrating, angry outbursts, or being hypervigilant.

Alcohol and tranquilizers are commonly abused by people with various anxiety disorders. These substances help decrease anxiety symptoms at first, but often lead to a dependency.

Psychotic Disorders

This category of mental illness is characterized by disturbances in the thought process.[23, 24] People suffering from *schizophrenia* have trouble telling the difference between reality and fantasy. The capacity to respond emotionally is also affected, and they may become withdrawn or unpredictable. People with this type of illness may hear voices, or have beliefs that don't make sense such as "others are out to get me," or "put thoughts in my mind." Some exhibit strange or unusual behaviors like talking to themselves in public or dressing in a very bizarre manner.

Personality Disorders

These involve ingrained traits that show in behaviors, leading to serious problems in life or a great deal of personal distress.[25, 26] These problems are usually repeated throughout life because the personality traits are so entrenched and hard to change.

There are many different types of personality disorders. Each involves a number of specific personality traits involving self-defeating behaviors that together, cause the person to feel a great deal of personal distress and/or have trouble getting along at work, school, home, or with others. Some problematic traits and behaviors associated with personality disorders include: strong mistrust of people, emotional coldness and aloofness, extreme self-centeredness, being overly dramatic, needing constant attention and admiration, lacking empathy or concern for others, being dishonest and lying, cheating or deceiving others, being unconcerned with the laws or rules of society, extreme shyness, impulsivity (acting before thinking), and excessive dependency.

Attention Deficit Disorder

These involve inattention and/or hyperactivity symptoms that are present for at least six months or longer and cause problems in your life.[27, 28] *Inattention* includes: failure to pay close attention to details and making careless mistakes (school, work, other activities); hard to keep paying attention to tasks or work; don't seem able to listen when others talk to you; failure to follow through with tasks (work, school, chores, instructions); difficulty organizing tasks or activities; avoiding activities that require you to keep paying attention; often losing things needed to complete tasks or activities (tools, books, etc.); easily distracted; and often forgetful.

Hyperactivity includes often fidgeting or trouble sitting still; hard to remain seated (at school or work); feeling restless; difficulty engaging in activities quietly; often "on the go" like you are "driven by a motor;" talking too much; or impulsive (say things without thinking, hard awaiting your turn, often interrupting others).

Other Addictive or Compulsive Disorders

These involve compulsive gambling, overeating, sex, use of the Internet or other activities that are out of control. The person is unable to stop these behaviors despite the fact that they are causing problems. Oftentimes, the family may be aware of the problem, but denial prevents the person from seeing the addiction or asking for help. Many people have more than one type of addictive disorder. And, many also have other psychiatric conditions such as depressive illness or a personality disorder.

Co-Occurring Disorders (Substance Use and Psychiatric Disorders)

There are many relationships between substance use and mental health disorders.[29] Having a psychiatric illness increases the risk for an alcohol or drug problem. Likewise, having an alcohol or drug problem increases the risk of psychiatric illness. Alcohol and drug use sometimes makes existing psychiatric symptoms worse or causes new symptoms. For example, some patients end up in the psychiatric hospital after using drugs like cocaine, marijuana, or alcohol, which lead to becoming severely depressed, manic, psychotic, or suicidal. In some cases, the use of these substances makes patients stop taking medication for their psychiatric illness or stop counseling sessions. In other cases, alcohol or drug use made the medications for the psychiatric illness less effective or ineffective. If you take an anti-depressant or anti-psychotic medicine while using alcohol or other drugs it can raise or lower the level of medicine in your blood, thus altering the effectiveness of it. Your medicine just won't work like it should if you drink alcohol or take street drugs or other non-prescribed drugs.

Some people develop an alcohol or drug addiction before experiencing a psychiatric disorder. Others develop their addiction after an episode of psychiatric illness. Regardless of which of your disorders came first, you still have to address both. Otherwise, you won't recover.

Causes of Disorders

There is no one simple way to explain why you developed a psychiatric or addictive disorder. Try to accept your illnesses as "no fault" caused by a combination of factors working together. No one "chooses" to have bipolar illness, schizophrenia, alcoholism, cocaine addiction, or other disorders. Medical and social scientists who study psychiatric illness and addictive illness report that they may result from the following factors.[30–32]

Biological

Illnesses such as depression, bipolar disease, schizophrenia, and alcoholism run in families. Scientists believe some of us inherit a "predisposition" to develop certain illnesses. There may be something in our brain chemistry or other biological aspect of our bodies that make us predisposed to having an illness. Just as diabetes, hypertension, or other medical problems run in many families, so too do psychiatric and addictive disorders.

Many substances mimic the action of one or more of the transmitters (chemical messengers) in your brain. Over time, alcohol or drugs can "hijack" the limbic system (also called the "reward pathway") in your brain. The "feeling" caused by using these substances over and over can surpass that experienced by natural methods of gaining pleasure (for example, from accomplishments or achievements, sports, sexual experience or other experiences in life). The result is that you may have strong cravings for alcohol or drugs and continue to use despite the negative consequences. What this means is that although you may have chosen to use drugs or alcohol at first, over time your addiction takes control of your brain and influences your behavior. Studies using MRI brain scans show significant differences in a brain of a person using drugs like cocaine or methamphetamine and a brain not under the influence of these drugs.[33]

The acute and long-term effects of alcohol and drugs can also cause psychiatric symptoms such as depression. Medical and health problems contribute to psychiatric disorders as well, which in turn can impact on alcohol or drug use.

Psychological

Your beliefs about the world and yourself, how you think, your personality, the ways you cope with stress and problems, and how you act may impact on whether or not you experience a psychiatric illness or addiction. Some people react differently to life stresses or problems than others. This means that some of us are more likely to experience mental distress and develop a psychiatric illness or use alcohol or drugs to cope.

Environmental

Your family, community, living environment, and culture affect you as well. Any of these factors may in one way or another impact the development of a psychiatric illness or addiction. Some people are more apt to abuse alcohol or drugs or develop psychiatric problems as a result of these factors.

Problems Associated with Substance Use Disorders

Substance use disorders can cause or worsen problems in any area of life. Examples of potential negative effects include the following problems.[34–35]

Medical or health related

These include increased risk of accidents, injuries or death; poor nutrition, increased risk of liver, heart, kidney or lung diseases, cancers of the mouth or pharynx; gastritis; dental problems; edema; high blood pressure; problems with sexual performance; complications with menstrual cycle, pregnancy or childbirth for women; increased risk of sexually transmitted diseases, hepatitis, HIV or AIDS; and premature death from the chronic effects of alcohol or drug use. Poor sleep or health habits (exercise, eating, getting regular dental or physical exams) are common, too.

Psychological or emotional

Examples include increased risk of anxiety, depression, mood swings, suicidal thoughts or actions, psychosis, poor control of impulses and behaviors, feelings of guilt and shame, low self-esteem, violence toward self or others and poor coping behaviors for dealing with stress, problems or upsetting emotions.

Family and children

Negative effects on the family include lost or damaged relationships due to separation or divorce; involvement in child welfare agencies; family distress and conflict; damaged relationships with family members, emotional burden for the family (anger, hurt, mistrust, fear, worry, depression), financial problems, poor communication and loss of respect; children are at increased risk for anxiety, depression, conduct disorders or other mental health problems, alcohol or drug abuse, or academic problems.

Interpersonal and social

Lost or damaged relationships, conflicts with others, dissatisfaction in intimate relationships, loss of trust or respect from others, or verbal or physical abuse; involvement with high risk people who drag you down, stopping or cutting down leisure activities not involving alcohol or drugs, or loss of interest in normal social activities.

Spiritual

Many people in recovery report the spiritual pain associated with addiction is worse than other types of pain. Negative effects on spirituality include feeling guilty, shameful or empty, loss of or less involvement in faith or religious practices, decline in moral values, disconnection from God or Higher Power, lack of meaning in life.

Occupational or academic

Some of the common problems in these areas include poor performance, loss of job, under-employment, unemployment, missing work or school, bad work or study habits, loss of motivation to succeed, ruined career, lost opportunities, dropping out of school or inability to manage work or school responsibly.

Economic

Insufficient or loss of income, inability to pay for basic needs (food, shelter, clothing, health care), excessive debt, loan defaults, ignoring financial obligations, loss of security or living arrangements, or poor money management are some of the common economic problems that may be caused or worsened by a substance use disorder.

Effects of Co-Occurring Disorders

Individuals with co-occurring disorders, especially those with chronic mental disorders, experience higher rates of:[36, 37]

- Disability, more days spent in the hospital, and more emergency room visits
- Poor treatment adherence and early drop out
- Relapse to either disorder; psychiatric hospitalization
- Medical problems including HIV infection and sexually transmitted diseases
- Family, social, occupational, and legal problems; violence and incarceration

The Importance of a Thorough Assessment

Assessment is used to determine your diagnoses and recommend the correct level of care such as inpatient, rehabilitation or outpatient. Assessment helps determine the type of treatments and services that you need such as therapy, medications, case management or a combination. Since the effects of alcohol and drugs can "mimic," cover-up, trigger off, or exaggerate any psychiatric symptom, you may need to be off alcohol and drugs for a couple weeks or longer before an accurate diagnosis can be given. You can help the assessment process by being totally honest about your symptoms and your alcohol and drug use patterns. If you hold back information about your substance use this can actually harm you as your caregivers may not be able to provide the treatment you need. Remember, they are out to help you, not judge you for what you have used.

A good assessment involves one or more interviews with professionals who ask questions about psychiatric symptoms, alcohol and drug use, medical, personal and family history. Your assessment may also involve a physical examination, lab tests and breathalyzer or urinalysis tests to determine what drugs are in your system or whether or not there are medical conditions caused by alcohol or drug use. Psychological tests may be used as well. Your assessment may involve filling out "self-reports" or written questionnaires. If you are physically addicted to alcohol or drugs like opioids, benzodiazepine (benzo) or barbiturates and undergoing evaluation for detoxification, your doctor and nurse may use withdrawal scales to determine what medicine you need, how much of it you need and how often. While in some cases assessment goes fairly smoothly, in other cases it is complex and takes time. Make sure you find out your diagnoses from the professionals who evaluate you.

The more you understand your diagnoses, the more you will understand what treatment can help you and what steps you can take to help yourself. You may be asked to involve your family or significant others in assessment and treatment. They can provide useful information to your treatment team. And, they may be a source of help and support to you. Treatment can help families understand their own feelings and reactions as well. Sometimes, other family members may need their own treatment for a psychiatric or addiction problem. Of course, it is ultimately up to you whether or not to involve your family or other significant people in your treatment. If you have reservations about involving others in your assessment or treatment, discuss these with your treatment team.

3. Treatment of Co-Occurring Disorders

Approaches to Treatment

There are three approaches to treatment of co-occurring disorders.[1, 2] The first, *sequential* treatment, involves getting your most acute or severe disorder treated first in one treatment program, then going to another program for the treatment of your other disorder. This sequential approach requires you to attend treatment in two different kinds of systems—mental health and drug and alcohol programs. It also requires authorizations from your private or public insurance company that pays for your care.

The second approach, *parallel,* involves getting your mental health disorder treated in a mental health program while at the same time getting your addictive disorder treated in a drug and alcohol program. This requires you to be involved in two separate treatment programs at the same time. It also requires authorizations from your insurance company.

The third approach, *integrated,* involves getting both of your disorders treated in the same program. Integrated treatment allows you to focus on both of your disorders by the same treatment team. While all three approaches can be helpful, the integrated approach is usually recommended, particularly in cases of more severe and chronic forms of psychiatric illness.[3–7]

Types of Treatment

A variety of time-limited and structured rehabilitation and treatment programs, individual, family, and group therapies and medications are used to treat co-occurring disorders. These services may be primarily focused on addiction, mental health disorders or both. The type of treatment offered will depend on your current problems and symptoms, your interest in treatment and motivation and what services are available in the treatment system you are engaged in.

Levels of Care

There are several levels of care for addiction, psychiatric or co-occurring disorders. You may move back and forth between these levels, depending on your current psychiatric symptoms, alcohol and drug use and problems created by your disorders. Levels of care from the least to most restrictive include:

Outpatient (OPT)

You meet regularly (weekly or less often) with a treatment group and/or individual therapist to discuss your current problems, symptoms, and concerns. OPT helps you focus on learning to manage your disorders and improve your coping skills. In some cases, it serves as "aftercare" for individuals discharged from inpatient or residential care.

Intensive Outpatient (IOP)

This is a structured group program, several hours per session, several days per week, usually for 4–12 weeks or longer. IOP services include recovery education and skill groups as well as therapy groups that allow members to discuss their specific problems. Individual therapy, medication management, and family therapy sessions are also offered in IOP.

Partial Hospital (PH)

Acute PH or day programs are usually offered four or more hours per day, up to seven days a week, for 2–4 weeks or longer. A PH is sometimes used as an alternative to hospitalization or as a "step-down" from inpatient care. The focus in PH care is to stabilize from the acute symptoms of your disorder, and learn ways to manage your disorders.

Non-Hospital Residential

These include both short-term (less than 90 days, although most rehabs are less than 28 days) and long-term (over 90 days) rehabilitation, halfway house and therapeutic community programs for the treatment of addiction, mental health disorders, or co-occurring disorders. Some programs are not integrated and it isn't unusual for people living in community-based residential addiction programs to attend a partial hospital or intensive outpatient program during the day for help with co-occurring psychiatric disorders.

Psychiatric Rehabilitation Programs

These are designed for individuals with chronic forms of disorders such as schizophrenia or bipolar illness. They involve a number of different types of groups and therapies such as education about illness, managing psychiatric symptoms, learning job preparation skills, improving communication and social skills and problem solving. These programs may last weeks or months. Individual therapy and sessions with the doctor for medication management are also offered in these programs.

Hospital Programs

These include short-term, acute care psychiatric, addiction detoxification and addiction rehabilitation programs that are medically managed. Acute care in a psychiatric hospital may last a few days to a few weeks. Medical detoxification from addictive substances is usually two to five days and usually is followed by a rehab program. Longer term care psychiatric hospital stays may last months or longer. The current trend is to stabilize individuals as quickly as possible and return them to the community so they can continue treatment in a partial hospital, intensive outpatient or outpatient program.

What to Expect from Treatment

Treatment should help eliminate or reduce your psychiatric symptoms, help you learn to manage your disorders, and help you deal with problems contributing to or resulting from your disorders. Treatment can also help you stop using alcohol or other drugs. Sessions with a therapist or doctor provide you a chance to talk about your symptoms, problems, coping strategies, and steps you can take to help yourself. You can disclose your inner thoughts and feelings, and gain a greater understanding of yourself and what you can do to change.

While there are many benefits to treatment, it can't solve all of your problems. If you have a chronic or persistent form of psychiatric illness, you may always experience some symptoms and distress. All chronic disorders (physical, mental, or addictive) require the capacity to learn to live with some degree of discomfort associated with symptoms that may never totally go away.

To get the most out of treatment, ask your therapist or counselor to give you feedback on how you are doing. Ask for recommendations on issues to work on. Also, be sure to talk about any problems or concerns you have about your therapist and how he or she works with you. If you have a problem with your caregiver, face it head-on rather than stop treatment because you raise your risk of relapse if you drop out early.

How to Benefit from Your Treatment

You will benefit from treatment only to the degree that you put forth time and effort, and work hard. To get the most from treatment take an active role, attend your sessions, take medications only as prescribed, learn to trust your caregivers, involve your family (or significant other) and use the support of others in recovery by attending mutual support programs.

Take an active role

Work with your treatment team to identify your problems, goals for treatment and develop a treatment plan. If you are unhappy with your treatment plan, discuss this with your therapist to see if any changes are needed. Although therapists, doctors, other professionals, and medications can help your recovery, you play a role in whether or not you get well and manage your illness. Taking responsibility and working hard to change and deal with your problems puts you in a position to get the most from treatment.

Attend all your sessions and take your medications only as prescribed

The biggest barrier to recovery and getting well is poor compliance with treatment.[8] If you miss your treatment sessions, don't take medications as prescribed, mix drugs or alcohol with your medicine, or fail to follow through with your treatment plan you decrease the chances of getting well. Individuals who comply with treatment usually do better than those who drop out early. Poor compliance with medications or therapy can increase your risk of relapse and hospitalization.

Develop a connection with your therapist and treatment team

This means you have to open up and trust the people caring for you and develop an alliance with them. Share your problems, feelings, and struggles. View your caregivers as "partners" in helping you understand and manage your co-occurring disorders. Report your progress and relapses to them so they can celebrate your successes with you as well as help you during rough times.

Involve your family or significant other in your treatment and recovery

You can involve your family or live-in partner in your treatment as well. Those close to you can benefit from learning about co-occurring disorders and recovery, what they can and can't do to help you, and what they can do to help themselves. Talk with them and your therapist about how they can get involved in your treatment and mutual support programs available to them.

Attend mutual support programs

There are many programs like Alcoholics Anonymous (AA), Narcotics Anonymous (NA), Dual Recovery Anonymous (DRA) other Twelve-Step, and non-Twelve-Step programs to aid recovery from addiction or co-occurring disorders. Programs like Recovery International and others can aid recovery from psychiatric illness. Support programs expose you to others recovering from similar disorders who can support you, teach you the ropes of recovery and be available to help during difficult times.

Other Services

Treatment programs can provide or refer you to other services for medical, housing, economic, social, school, work, spiritual or nutritional problems or needs. For example, case managers can help you access services you need to address other problems interfering with your ability to participate in professional treatment. Faith-based professionals can provide you spiritual guidance. Vocational counselors can help assess your vocational abilities, needs, and help you develop a plan if needed. If you continue to get high on alcohol or drugs, you can sabotage your chances of getting some of these services or benefiting from them. Always keep in mind that sobriety is important and gives you the maximum opportunity to take advantage of other services and programs.

Treatment Outcome

Many studies show that treatment is effective for psychiatric illness, addiction, or co-occurring disorders.[9–12] You can experience positive effects of treatment even if all of your symptoms don't go away, you still have problems in your life, or you relapse to either of your disorders. Remember, progress is relative—improvement in any area of your life, no matter how small, is a sign of progress. Quality of life often improves as a result of treatment. Positive effects of treatment may include:

- Stopping alcohol or drug use or reducing the amount or frequency of use.

- Remission or reduced severity of psychiatric symptoms.

- Better mental, physical or spiritual health.

- Improved social, family, financial, and occupational functioning.

- Better quality of life.

SECTION II

Setting the Foundation
for Recovery

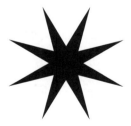

4. Why I Came to Treatment

One of the first important tasks of recovery is to identify the symptoms and problems that led you to treatment for your co-occurring disorders. In early recovery, the focus is mainly on stabilizing your symptoms and figuring out your longer-term recovery plan. Following is a brief list of some of the more common symptoms of psychiatric disorders and addiction that cause people to come to a treatment program.

Recovery Activity

1. Check the problems and symptoms that led to or caused you to come to treatment at this time.
   - ☐ Depression: sadness, loss of interest in life, hard to concentrate, low energy, poor appetite or sleep, feeling hopeless about future, suicidal thoughts or feelings

   - ☐ Mania: euphoric mood, mood swings, racing thoughts, high activity level

   - ☐ Self-harm: cutting or burning self, overdosing on pills, suicide attempt

   - ☐ Violent thoughts, plans or actions toward others

   - ☐ Suicidal thoughts, plans, or attempt

   - ☐ Psychotic symptoms: hearing voices (hallucinations), strange thoughts (delusions), feeling paranoid, out of touch with reality, confused, agitated

   - ☐ Severe or persistent anxiety and worry

   - ☐ Avoiding situations that cause anxiety

   - ☐ Severe panic attacks

   - ☐ Excessive fears or phobias (leaving home, flying, closed spaces, heights)

   - ☐ Obsessive thoughts (repeating things over and over in my mind)

   - ☐ PTSD: recurrent and distressing thoughts of a past trauma

   - ☐ Compulsive rituals: counting, checking, hoarding

   - ☐ Alcohol abuse or addiction

   - ☐ Cocaine abuse or addiction

   - ☐ Opioid abuse or addiction (heroin, pain pills, or narcotics)

   - ☐ Other drug abuse or addiction (nicotine, marijuana, benzos, other pills)

   - ☐ Other compulsions: gambling, sex, eating, spending, use of Internet, other

   - ☐ Serious problems with my spouse, partner or other family member or friends

   - ☐ Unable to take care of myself

   - ☐ Quit taking my psychiatric medication and got sick

   - ☐ Quit taking medications for opioid or alcohol addiction and relapsed

- ❏ Quit going to treatment and got sick with psychiatric symptoms or relapsed
- ❏ Difficulty controlling anger or bad temper problems
- ❏ In trouble with the law
- ❏ Had no place to live, ran out of money, life is a mess
- ❏ I was involuntarily committed to treatment
- ❏ I was pressured by my family to get help
- ❏ I was encouraged or pressured by the legal system (parole/probation), a social service agency, or my employer to get help

2. Discuss why you are in treatment at this time. _____

_____

_____

_____

_____

3. Describe what you think caused your psychiatric disorder. _____

_____

_____

_____

_____

4. Describe what you think caused your alcohol or drug problem. _____

_____

_____

_____

_____

Example #1: Anthony's Reasons for Coming to the Hospital

"I was doing good for a while. Then, I missed my counseling sessions and ran out of medications. Since I was feeling good, I quit treatment thinking I didn't need it any longer. In a few weeks I got real down. I couldn't shake it so I drank and used drugs again, thinking this would help my mood. All it did was make me worse. Got more depressed. When I went back to the crack pipe, I didn't care what happened to me. Wasn't important if I lived or died. That's how desperate I felt before coming to the hospital. I know now I gotta get back on track. Get clean and stay clean, and stay in treatment for my depression. I can't stop my medication unless my doctor tells me to."

Example #2: Kim's Reasons for Seeking Outpatient Treatment

"I can't seem to stay away from the alcohol. I get a few months sober then drink again. I feel nervous and depressed almost all of the time and can't get rid of my obsessive thoughts. I know this sometimes leads me to drinking, which then drives my friends away because of how I treat them. They tell me I'm too intense and demanding. I don't know how to have a good relationship and hook up with the wrong kind of guy. I need help with a lot of things, not just my drinking. Treatment helped me in the past and I hope it helps me again."

5. My Alcohol and Drug History

The first step in getting clean or sober is admitting that you have a problem with alcohol or other drugs. One of the ways you can do this is to take a close look at your alcohol and drug use and how it has affected your life. Answer the following questions about your alcohol and drug use. Share your answers with a counselor, an AA, NA, or CA sponsor, or other trusted person.

1. In the past 90 days how many days have you used?
    Alcohol _____
    Marijuana or hash _____
    Cocaine or crack _____
    Stimulants (speed, meth, uppers) _____
    Opiates, narcotics, pain pills _____
    Tranquilizers or downers _____
    Hallucinogens or acid _____
    Inhalants: glues, aerosols, etc. _____
    PCP or angel dust _____
    Other drugs (write in) _____
    How many years have you been using alcohol? _____
    How many years have you been using other drugs? _____
    I've gotten high on drugs or alcohol too many times to count. ❏ Yes ❏ No

2. I've experienced the following symptoms or behaviors related to alcohol or drug use:
    - ❏ **Excessive or inappropriate use of alcohol or other drugs:** getting high or drunk and not being able to fulfill my obligations at home, work, or with others; or feeling like I need substances to fit in with others or to function at work or home; driving under the influence of alcohol or drugs; using alcohol to help me come down off drugs; using drugs so I can drink more alcohol or party longer; overdosing on drugs.
    - ❏ **Changes in tolerance:** needing more alcohol or drugs to get high; getting high much easier or with less alcohol or drugs than I used in the past.
    - ❏ **Withdrawal symptoms:** getting physically sick when I cut down or stop using (for example, having the shakes, feeling nauseous, having gooseflesh, having a runny nose); experiencing mental symptoms such as depression, anxiety, or agitation.
    - ❏ **Using alcohol or drugs to avoid or stop withdrawal symptoms:** using substances regularly to avoid withdrawal sickness; drinking or using drugs to stop oncoming withdrawal symptoms; drinking in the morning to stop the shakes.
    - ❏ **Having trouble cutting down or stopping once I drink or take drugs:** not being able to control how much or how often I use; using more alcohol or drugs than I planned or for longer than intended.
    - ❏ **Stopping my use for a period of time only to go back again:** staying sober for a while then relapsing.
    - ❏ **Spending a great deal of time in activities to get substances, use them or recover from their effects:** my use of substances or their effects may consume much of my time.

❑ **Giving up important activities or losing friendships because of my use:** stopping activities that were once important to me; giving up friends who don't get high; losing friends because of the way my alcohol and drug use affects my behavior with others.

❑ **Continuing to use alcohol or other drugs even though they cause problems:** ignoring the advice of my doctor, therapist, or other professional to stop using because of the problems substances have caused; using again even though I know this causes medical, emotional, family, work, legal, financial, or spiritual problems.

Write in the number of addiction symptoms that you checked off: _____

If you checked three or more symptoms, you have a dependency (addiction) problem. If you checked one or two, you still have a problem that is likely to interfere with your psychiatric recovery if you don't do something about it.

3. Which of the following *high-risk behaviors* have you ever engaged in?
    ❑ Shooting drugs with a needle
    ❑ Sharing needles, cotton, or rinsing water with others; using unsterile needles
    ❑ Smoking crack, meth or freebase cocaine
    ❑ Overdosing on drugs
    ❑ Going to "shooting galleries" or "crack houses" to get high
    ❑ Lying to doctors, nurses, or dentists in order to get drugs
    ❑ Going to a hospital emergency room and faking symptoms to get drugs
    ❑ Trading sex for alcohol or drugs, or to get money for substances
    ❑ Having high risk sex (with strangers or multiple partners with no protection)
    ❑ Drinking mouthwash or other products for the alcohol content
    ❑ Committing crimes to get money for alcohol or drugs
    ❑ Committing crimes as a result of effects of alcohol or drugs on my judgment
    ❑ Getting arrested as a result of using (DUI, public intoxication, etc.).

4. How would you rate the severity of your problem with alcohol or drugs?
    ❑ Mild problem
    ❑ Moderate problem
    ❑ Severe problem
    ❑ Life-threatening problem
    ❑ Not sure

5. How would you rate your need for treatment for your alcohol or other drug problem?
    ❑ Not sure if I need treatment
    ❑ I think I need treatment
    ❑ I definitely need treatment

6. From reviewing my completed checklist I would say this about my alcohol and drug problem.

_____
_____
_____
_____
_____
_____
_____
_____
_____
_____
_____
_____
_____
_____
_____
_____
_____

Example #1: Leroy's Review

"After thinking about my alcohol and drug use, I'd have to say my addiction has kicked my ass real good. I've been getting high on booze and dope for a long time, too many years to count. OD'd a couple of times, lied, cheated, scammed, stole, lost jobs. You name it, I did it to cop some shit. Ain't no doubt about it, my addiction is bad. Been a big factor in going to jail and going in and out of detox centers and psychiatric hospitals."

Example #2: Gail's Review

"Until recently I never considered myself an addict because I didn't use street drugs. All I used was alcohol and pills I got from a doctor. Many, many pills. Got them from a couple of doctors. I lied about my symptoms so I could get pills for back pain and bad nerves. I didn't think I was addicted because doctors gave me these pills. The reason I never made much progress before with my psychiatric problem was I kept taking so many pills. To recover, I have to stop lying to get pills and learn to deal with pain and anxiety without relying on drugs."

6. Effects of Disorders on My Life

Co-occurring disorders can affect any area of your life. This includes your physical health, your relationships with family, friends and co-workers, your ability to take care of your basic needs, and your overall adjustment and happiness. An important part of early recovery is taking a look at the effects of your co-occurring disorders on your life. Although this can cause you some anxiety at first, it can help motivate you to work hard at your recovery.

In your own words, state how you think either or both of your disorders affected different areas of your life. There may be an overlap in some of these areas.

Physical health (including medical and dental problems)

_____

_____

Diet and eating habits

_____

_____

Sexual desire or behavior

_____

_____

Exercise habits

_____

_____

Relationships with parents

_____

_____

Relationships with spouse or partner

_____

_____

Relationships with children, stepchildren, grandchildren

_____

_____

Relationships with boss or co-workers

_____

_____

Relationships with friends

_____

_____

Faith or spirituality

_____

_____

Work or school

_____

_____

Lost opportunities or wasted talents or abilities

_____

_____

Hobbies, leisure interests, or recreational habits

_____

_____

Financial condition

_____

_____

Difficulty with the law or other legal problems

_____

_____

Involvement in high-risk behaviors

_____

_____

Other problems

_____

_____

Summarize how your disorders have affected your life:

_____

_____

_____

_____

_____

_____

_____

Example #1: Sandra's Review

"Both my problems messed me up. My depression, cutting myself and getting into fights got me in trouble with the law. Plus, it made my kids upset. When I was at my worst, I thought about overdosing on drugs to end it all. Life just felt like shit and I didn't have nothing to live for. When I was shooting drugs, I didn't care who I got high with. It's a wonder I didn't get AIDS cause I shared needles. When I starting smoking crack, I sold sex for drugs and got hooked up with some nasty men. But I'd do anything to get my rocks to smoke. My addiction caused me to lose jobs. I couldn't take good care of my kids and almost lost them. I felt like a nobody. I feel I have a chance now to put my life back together."

Example #2: Paul's Review

"I thought long and hard about the effects of my alcoholism and anxiety. Drinking caused me to gain weight and ignore my health. I stopped exercising. I have a great job but came late or missed too many days. My anxiety and worry upset my wife and kids. In recent years I avoided getting together with people outside of the family because of my anxiety. This hurt my family, especially my wife who became frustrated because we didn't go out in public hardly at all. Even though I thought drinking calmed me down, it made my anxiety worse. I got caught up in a vicious cycle."

7. My Problem List and Strengths

In the space below, list the specific problems you need to work on first while in treatment. These should relate to the reasons you sought help on your own or were committed to treatment. This list should include both your psychiatric and your alcohol/drug-abuse disorders.

1. Psychiatric _____

   _____

   _____

2. Alcohol/Drug Abuse or Addiction _____

   _____

   _____

3. Family or Relationship _____

   _____

   _____

4. Other (e.g., legal, work, living arrangements) _____

   _____

   _____

Example #1: Russell's Problem List
1. Feeling depressed, not caring about my life or having any goals or direction.
2. Addiction to crack, alcohol and marijuana.
3. I was living with other addicts and need a sober living environment.
4. I got a short fuse and need to control my anger and rage.

Example #2: Juanita's Problem List
1. Being impulsive and dropping out of treatment when I feel better or don't like my counselor.
2. Alcohol and drug abuse and how it put a wedge between me and my children.
3. I'm a real nervous person who worries a lot and need to deal with this without getting high.
4. I have trouble keeping a job because I miss work and get fired or quit.

My Strengths

It is helpful in recovery to build on your strengths or positive qualities. Your strengths refer to things that are positive about yourself or your life. They include:

- Your positive qualities such as being kind, assertive, creative, hardworking, resilient, or open and honest with others.
- Your attitudes and motivation such as really wanting to stay sober and make things better in life, being committed to recovery, or wanting to get ahead in life.
- Your lifestyle such as having a job, having adequate money to take care of your needs, having leisure interests and hobbies that you enjoy, being organized, having goals that you are working toward.
- Your faith, religion or spiritual beliefs or knowing you are capable of change.
- Your relationships such as having family or friends that you are close to and who support and care about you.

List other strengths or positive aspects about yourself, your life, or relationships.

_____

_____

_____

_____

Example #1: Shawna's Strengths

1. I'm a good mother and like taking care of my kids. I give them lots of love and attention.
2. I don't give up easily. I work hard to get ahead and don't give up when things get tough.
3. I have a good sense of humor.
4. I'm motivated to change. I want to stay clean, get my life together and quit hurting others.
5. I don't mind asking for help. I'm willing to let my NA sponsor and therapist help me.

Example #2: Drew's Strengths

1. I am energetic and work hard.
2. People like me because I'm easy to talk with and get along with.
3. I have relationships with several close friends based on mutual respect and interests.
4. I'm grounded in my spiritual beliefs and am connected to the church.
5. I have lots of creative interests, which I enjoy and give me great satisfaction.

8. My Goals While I'm in Treatment

List the major symptoms of your psychiatric disorders and several steps you can take to manage (stop or reduce) these symptoms. Do the same for your alcohol or drug problem. When you list steps you will take, be as specific as you can.

Psychiatric disorder (list major symptoms of your disorder):

_____

_____

My goal(s) in relation to my psychiatric disorder (usually to stop or reduce symptoms):

(1) _____

_____

(2) _____

_____

Steps I can take to reach my goal(s) (specific actions you take to help yourself):

(1) _____

_____

(2) _____

_____

(3) _____

_____

(4) _____

_____

Alcohol or drug abuse or addiction (brief description of problem):

_____

_____

My goal(s) in relation to this problem (abstinence is highly recommended):

(1) _____

_____

(2) _____

_____

Steps I can take to reach my goal(s) (what you can do to get and stay sober):

(1) _____

_____

(2) _____

_____

(3) _____

_____

(4) _____

_____

Example #1: Maureen

Psychiatric Disorder: depression with low energy, hard to get moving, poor appetite, poor concentration, feelings of hopelessness, and feeling like life is passing me by. Sometimes I even wonder if life is worth living although I would not take my own life.

Goals: to reduce my depressed feelings and decrease the proportion of negative to positive thoughts that I have so that I feel better and can take care of my responsibilities.

Steps to Her Goals: follow a daily schedule to keep active, engage in at least one enjoyable activity each day, take antidepressants every day (don't skip doses), exercise for 30 minutes or more at least four days a week, eat regular meals, challenge negative thinking and replace it with more realistic thinking.

Example #2: Andy

Alcohol Problem: I became dependent on alcohol and drank heavily too often, which led to getting a drunk driving arrest, having blackouts, not taking care of my family responsibilities (ignored wife and kids) and worsened my mood.

Goals: to stop drinking and replace time spent drinking with healthy activities that keep me busy and bring me pleasure.

Steps to His Goals: go to my meetings (AA) three times a week, talk with my AA sponsor every day, use active strategies to fight off desires or cravings for alcohol, stay connected to others in recovery, and spend more time with my wife and our children.

9. My Motivation to Change

One of the challenges you face in recovery is to develop and maintain your motivation to change. At first, it isn't unusual to have mixed feelings about changing. One part of you wants to quit using substances, get help with your psychiatric disorder and change your life while another part of you may not want to change both problems. Motivation is not stable over time so be prepared for fluctuations in your motivation, especially in the first few months of recovery.

Researchers and clinicians have identified stages that people often go through when dealing with a problem such as alcohol or drug abuse or addiction, or a mental health problem.[1-3] One widely accepted approach to change involves the following phases.[4]

1. **Precontemplation:** you deny or minimize your problem or don't see any need to change.

2. **Contemplation:** you agree you have a problem and plan to change in the next several months.

3. **Preparation:** you plan to take action on your problem within the next month or so. You may let others know about your intention to change.

4. **Action:** you actually change by stopping your alcohol or drug use, or getting help for your substance use disorder or mental health problem.

5. **Maintenance:** you continue to focus on making changes in yourself and your lifestyle to reduce the chances of a future relapse to either of your disorders.

6. **Termination:** your problem is under control and you feel you have the skills and confidence to continue coping with your disorders.

Assessing Your Stage of Change

There is no one way that all people progress through these stages so they are meant as "rough" guidelines. You can assess where you are by answering the following questions.

1. Do you think you have a mental health problem?
    ❑ Definitely   ❑ Probably   ❑ I'm not sure   ❑ Definitely not

2. Do you think you have an alcohol or drug problem?
    ❑ Definitely   ❑ Probably   ❑ I'm not sure   ❑ Definitely not

3. Are you willing to make a commitment to address your disorders?
    ❑ Definitely   ❑ Probably   ❑ I'm not sure   ❑ Definitely not

4. Are you willing to participate in treatment to help you with your disorders?
    ❑ Definitely   ❑ Probably   ❑ I'm not sure   ❑ Definitely not

5. Are you willing to make a commitment to quit using alcohol or other drugs?
    ❑ Definitely   ❑ Probably   ❑ I'm not sure   ❑ Definitely not

6. Are you willing to actively participate in mutual support programs?
    ❑ Definitely   ❑ Probably   ❑ I'm not sure   ❑ Definitely not

7. Are you willing to keep your counseling appointments and take medications as prescribed to help you recover from your disorders?
    ❑ Definitely   ❑ Probably   ❑ I'm not sure   ❑ Definitely not

8. Do you know the relapse risk factors for both of your disorders?
   ❏ Definitely   ❏ Probably   ❏ I'm not sure   ❏ Definitely not

9. Do you have a plan to deal with your relapse risk factors and manage warning signs?
   ❏ Definitely   ❏ Probably   ❏ I'm not sure   ❏ Definitely not

Strategies to Strengthen Your Motivation to Change

1. Accept that low motivation is common, and that as long as you hang in there and follow your recovery plan, you can overcome periods of low motivation.

2. Review your reasons for making a commitment to recovery and changing yourself.

3. Identify benefits of staying sober and managing your psychiatric disorder.

4. Accept recovery as a "we" program involving the support of others.

5. Share your motivational struggles with others in recovery, such as a sponsor, other members of mutual support programs, a counselor or someone you trust.

6. Find out what others in recovery did to strengthen their motivation to change.

7. Keep up your recovery disciplines even when you don't feel like it such as: going to meetings and counseling, reading, praying, using self-talk or meditating.

8. Remember the problems and negative aspects of alcohol or other drug use.

9. Read recovery or inspirational literature (or listen to audiobooks).

10. Advantages of Recovery

Giving up alcohol and drugs, and getting involved in recovery from co-occurring disorders takes time, effort and work. At first, it may be difficult to imagine what it will be like to live without using alcohol or other drugs. Assessing the advantages and disadvantages of giving up substances and staying involved in recovery can help your efforts to change.

Recovery Activity

1. List the advantages and disadvantages of stopping your use of alcohol or other drugs. Think of both short-term and long-term advantages.

Advantages	Disadvantages

2. List the advantages and disadvantages of staying involved in recovery from co-occurring disorders.

Advantages	Disadvantages

Good-bye Letter

Imagine that you could say anything you wanted to your alcohol or drug problems in a good-bye letter. In the space below, write a letter, expressing all of your feelings about what substance problem has done to you, and what it will be like to live without alcohol or other drugs.

Dear Alcohol or Drug Problem:

_____

_____

_____

_____

_____

_____

_____

_____

_____

_____

_____

_____

_____

_____

_____

_____

_____

_____

_____

_____

_____

_____

_____

_____

_____

_____

_____

11. Medical and Psychiatric Effects of My Drug and Alcohol Problem

Drug and alcohol use and a chaotic lifestyle can cause or worsen medical, dental and mental health problems. Existing problems can worsen or new problems may develop due to:

- The direct effects of substances on your body
- Accidents caused by being under the influence of substances
- Your diet and health care habits
- Impurities in drugs
- Complications caused by mixing drugs or using drugs and alcohol together
- Complications caused by using dirty needles to inject drugs, snorting or smoking drugs
- Engaging in high risk behaviors (unprotected sex, driving under the influence, violence, etc.)
- Your overall lifestyle

Alcohol and drugs can cause, worsen, or mask psychiatric symptoms, or contribute to relapse. Alcohol and drugs often interfere with recovery from psychiatric illness.

Recovery Activity

Answer the following questions regarding the effects of alcohol and drug use on your medical or mental health.

1. As a result of my alcohol or drug use, I've experienced:
    - ❑ An injury from an accident (home, work, car, boat, etc.)
    - ❑ Anxiety
    - ❑ Blackouts (periods of time I can't remember)
    - ❑ Close to death experience
    - ❑ Dental cavities, loss of teeth, poor hygiene, other problems
    - ❑ Depression
    - ❑ Diet problems (poor diet, don't follow special diet, etc.)
    - ❑ Digestive system complications (ulcer, gastritis, pancreatitis)
    - ❑ Emotional turmoil or poor control of emotions
    - ❑ Frequent headaches, bouts with the flu, or generally feeling sick
    - ❑ Frequent visits to doctors, clinics, hospitals, or emergency rooms
    - ❑ Hearing voices (hallucinations) or unusual beliefs (delusions)
    - ❑ Heart pain, heart attack, heart muscle damage
    - ❑ Infectious diseases (Hepatitis, HIV or AIDS, STDs, TB)
    - ❑ Mania (high moods)
    - ❑ Overdose of drugs
    - ❑ Poor eating or health care habits

- ❑ Pregnancy while addicted to alcohol or drugs (affecting developing baby)
- ❑ Psychiatric problems
- ❑ Seizures or convulsions
- ❑ Sex with strangers, multiple partners or with no protection (risky behaviors)
- ❑ Sexual problems (difficulty performing, loss of interest)
- ❑ Weight gain or loss of ten pounds or more (unintentional)
- ❑ Withdrawal sickness when I cut down or stopped using chemicals
- ❑ Worsening of other medical or psychiatric conditions (e.g., diabetes, depression)

2. Other problems that I've experienced include: _____
_____
_____

3. The last time that I had a physical examination was: _____

4. The last time that I had a dental examination was: _____

5. Describe your exercise habits: _____
_____
_____

Example: Richard's Goal

"I used to be a good athlete until drugs got the best of me causing medical problems. I lost a lot of weight and became run down. My first goal is to get my health back. I can do this by staying off drugs and not drinking alcohol since booze always leads me back to drugs. Been fooling myself too long about the alcohol. I'm also following a routine now so I can get enough rest and sleep at night. I'm going to bed at the same time each night and getting up at the same time. I'm eating decent meals at regular times. Plus, I'm exercising at least four days each week to get in shape. I need this discipline to get my health and self-respect back."

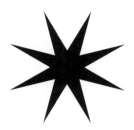

SECTION III

Accepting Your Disorders and Developing a Recovery Plan

12. Denial

This section will help you understand denial, how it relates to your disorders, and why it's critical to work through it in order to recover. Try to relate the material and stories to your life as much as possible. Talk about your questions, concerns, and reactions with your therapist or other helping professional, or a sponsor. Listen to what Lamont, Karen, Bill, and Lisa say about their substance use or psychiatric problems. See what you can learn about denial from them.

Ain't Nobody's Business What I Do

"All my running people get high. It's the thing to do. Ain't no big thing, really, getting high on crack. Don't do it every day. You'd do it too if you lived in my neighborhood. Shit, it really ain't nobody's business what I do. What I do is on me and I'm tellin' you man, I like to get high.

Yeah, I got busted by the cops. But hey, they had it in for me. Got a bad break, that's all. My PO makes me go to these meetings and get slips signed. Gotta go to counseling too and piss in a bottle. That MF don't know shit cause he ain't never been where I am. Talking about me being an addict and shit just because I smoke some rocks."—*Lamont, age 27*

I Like to Get High

"OK, so I like to get high. I've been getting high since I was 14. I enjoy getting loaded. Taking drugs makes me relax and feel mellow. I'm a real nervous type of person, but drugs help calm me down. I don't use needles or "hard" stuff like heroin or cocaine. Believe me, there's a lot of people worse off than me. I don't think that drugs affect my work. I have a job and hardly ever miss work. In fact, I just got a raise. I don't ever use when I visit my parents and they've never seen me loaded. And, drugs don't affect my relationships. Most of my friends like to get high, too. I'm not hurting anyone else. I have a right to get high if I want to. If drugs really get out of hand, then I'll probably quit. But for now, I just don't want to stop."—*Karen, age 34*

What's Wrong with Feeling So Good?

"I've always been an energetic person. I like working a lot and being involved in life. I can't help it if I don't need much sleep and get up early in the morning. What's wrong with being on the go all the time and wanting to accomplish things? Everyone is so negative these days. I want to be a positive person and get things done. You can't sleep your whole life away. It's a drag when you're not active and it gets real boring. There's just so much to do.

My wife and sponsor think I need to see a shrink. What do they know about me? I think they are jealous because I feel so good and accomplish so much. They need to take their own inventory and not mine, and stay out of my business. What's so wrong with feeling so good, like you can do anything at all? After all, I'm making lots of extra money because I can work so many hours. Besides, I like feeling on top of the world. And, why should my wife get on me for spending money. After all, I'm making good money so why can't I spend a few hundred here and there. My wife is upset because I bought some golf clubs. I've always wanted to play golf so what's the big damn deal? My wife is also upset because I bought some stock with the kids' college money. Hey, I found some good stocks and I know I'll make a killing and probably triple their money.

These people keep bugging me, especially my wife. She also accuses me of snapping out at her and the kids and being unreasonable. What can I say? If the kids mess up, I'm just going to tell them and get on them to clean up their acts. What's so unreasonable about this? Can't a father discipline his kids without his wife butting in? She should talk, because I've heard her get on the kids many times. I'm just going to keep on doing what I've been doing. Work hard, stay active, and look for opportunities to make money. I know I can make a bundle. Everyone wants to get rich, don't they?"—*Bill, age 42*

I Should Be Able to Pull Myself Up

"I've been clean from dope for almost eight months now and don't understand why I'm depressed. There's no reason why I shouldn't be able to pull myself out of this. My therapist and doctor want me to take medications for depression. But I kicked a big dope habit and have been clean eight months. I used every day for a couple of years. If I can kick my heroin addiction, there's no reason why I can't shake my depression. I want to be totally clean and off all drugs. I'll just keep working and pull myself out of this. After all, I'm a strong woman. I think if you can stop shooting dope, you should be able to do anything."—*Lisa, age 29*

Many people like Lamont, Karen, Bill, and Lisa experience problems because of their drinking or drug use, their psychiatric illness, or both. Yet many deny their alcohol or drug use is a problem or that they have a psychiatric disorder. Some even deny both disorders. Why do they do this?

Denial is a refusal to believe or accept some reality in your life. It's a "defense mechanism" that occurs without your being aware of it. It happens unconsciously and "protects" you from anxiety that comes from facing the truth about having a serious problem such as an addiction or psychiatric disorder. Denial prevents many people with alcohol or drug problems from seeking help. It is considered the "fatal aspect" of the disease of addiction because the end result of untreated addiction may be an early death or some other serious consequence.

Denial also prevents many people with psychiatric disorders from seeking help. As a result, many continue to suffer with their symptoms or continue to act in ways that interfere with their well-being or happiness. Some only get help as a result of an involuntary commitment.

Examples of Denial

You may deny your psychiatric illness, your addiction, or both. You may deny one disorder by blaming your problems on the other. As you review the following list of how denial shows, make a note of which ones you relate to.

- Not believing you have a problem with alcohol or drug use despite evidence to the contrary.
- Minimizing your alcohol and drug use, and believing "it's not that bad." Others use more stuff, or more often than you.
- Blaming difficulties on "other" problems (e.g., boss, spouse, friends, pressures, mental illness) and not your substance use.
- Believing you can "cut down" and limit how much or how often you use, especially if you get help with your psychiatric disorder.
- Believing that since you are giving up your main drug of abuse, you can still use other substances (i.e., giving up crack but drinking alcohol or smoking pot).
- Thinking that since you don't use large quantities, don't use every day, or don't get loaded every time that you use, you can't have a serious drug or alcohol problem.

- Thinking you can't be hooked because you don't suffer physical withdrawal symptoms when you cut down or stop using, or don't always "crave" alcohol or drugs.

- Believing after a period of sobriety and recovery that your problem is "under control" and you can "handle" a few drinks (pills, tokes, lines, etc.).

- Saying that you can't have a problem because you hold a job, take care of your family, haven't gotten into major difficulties, or don't act "crazy."

- Believing that no one else has been affected by your addiction or psychiatric problems.

- Blaming your psychiatric symptoms and problems on your use of alcohol or other drugs.

- Believing that if you stop using alcohol or drugs, your psychiatric disorder will improve.

- Blaming your psychiatric problems on bad luck, bad breaks, or bad friends.

The cases cited earlier show examples of denial in relation to addiction and psychiatric disorders. Lamont got busted by the cops and was forced to go to NA and counseling, but didn't think smoking crack was a problem. Karen denied that she had a problem because she didn't use "hard stuff" like heroin or cocaine, and didn't think her drug use affected her life in any negative ways. In fact, she saw drugs as "helping" her because it reduced her anxiety. Bill didn't admit that anything was wrong with him despite the fact that his manic behavior became increasingly worse. And, Lisa minimized her depression, particularly since she felt she should be able to "pull herself up."

To other people, denial of addiction may come across as willful lying or conning. Others usually see your situation more clearly than you do because your judgment is impaired by your substance use, or you have blackouts and don't remember being loaded, or the things you said or did while under the influence.

Denial of your psychiatric disorder may come across to others as poor judgment on your part. They may wonder why you can't see that you have a psychiatric problem. Your illness itself can contribute to denial.

Family and Societal Denial

Family members can deny or minimize the effects of either or both of your co-occurring disorders. They may not want to believe or accept the reality that you are an alcoholic or drug addict, or have a psychiatric illness. It may bring too much shame or embarrassment upon them. With co-occurring disorders some families may blame all of your troubles on your addiction and refuse to accept that you also have a psychiatric disorder. Or, they may accept that you have a psychiatric illness and deny that your alcohol or drug use has anything to do with your difficulties.

The Effects of Denial

Many people with co-occurring disorders never get help or don't get the correct help because of their denial. As a result, they experience negative consequences. The following comments show different effects of denial of addiction, psychiatric disorders or both:

"Everybody knew I was messed up on crack. Everybody but me, that is. I stole, lied, conned, scammed, cheated and ripped people off to get money for some rocks. It was an everyday thing. My woman left me and told me she didn't want nothing to do with me unless I stopped getting high. Even my momma told me to straighten my ass out and get off the crack cause it was messing with my mind. Got popped by my PO for violating my probation but I still didn't think my drug use was that bad. Crack made me lose everything, even my freedom, before I saw it as my addiction."

—*Tony, age 26*

"I prescribed myself drugs to feel better and control my anxiety. Then I started using cocaine. Even though things got real bad, I still used drugs. After all, I'm a doctor and know what's best for me. I continued to deny my drug addiction until I lost my license to practice medicine. My husband left me and my life was shattered. I felt guilty and shameful and very depressed. My life had no meaning. It took a while, but I finally rebounded and put my life back together. But only after I got help for both my addiction and depression."—*Kelli, age 35*

"Everyone knew I was an alcoholic. Yet I continued to deny it. I drank heavily my whole life. It messed up my family and my health. Some friends ditched me because of how I acted. It wasn't until I suffered with gastritis and my doctor convinced me to get help that I got help."—*Matt, age 57*

"I quit or lost a lot of jobs because my panic and anxiety symptoms caused me to miss a lot of work. I became undependable. I lied to cover my tracks but this didn't work. I often told myself I was getting bad breaks, that this was the reason for my job problems. Until I accepted that I had a mental problem and got help I wasn't able to break this pattern."—*Amy, age 41*

"I lost my daddy to drugs. He told us to quit bugging him about drugs, that he had things under control. He just wouldn't stop. I really miss him. Why did he have to die from taking drugs?"

—*Lauren, age 12*

"My wife and daughter kept telling me that I needed help when my mood became real high, but I ignored them. As my mania got worse, I did crazier things. I really hurt my family and put my job in jeopardy. But I was lucky and finally got forced to get help before I lost everything."

—*Ron, age 39*

"I've always had psychiatric problems and had no trouble admitting these. But addiction? No way. I used alcohol and drugs to have fun, calm me down, or make my hallucinations go away. Then, I'd stop taking my medication which led to getting sicker. A couple times I ended up back in the psych hospital. It was only after I finally admitted to my addiction that I started to get better. Since being straight for over nine months, my schizophrenia isn't as bad."—*Becka, age 21*

"I was a con long before I got hooked on booze and drugs. I stole, cheated, lied, and took advantage of everyone I could. Used women for whatever I could get from them. Wasn't nobody important to me and I only looked out for number one. Sold drugs and stolen property to support my lifestyle. I lived on the edge and got in a lot of fights. Got shot once and stabbed a couple times. Messed up too many people to count. Spent time in prison twice and mental institutions. Wasn't until I quit blaming society for my troubles and made a decision to get clean and stop this crazy shit that things changed. My problems messed me up for a lot of years."—*Carlton, age 29*

These brief quotes show a variety of the effects of denial. Many medical, emotional, social, family, financial, legal, and spiritual problems are caused by denying one or both of your co-occurring disorders.

Why Deny Your Disorder?

The effects of alcohol or drugs can contribute to your denial. For example, you may feel good after drinking alcohol, feel energized after snorting cocaine or smoking crack, or feel mellow after smoking pot or taking an opiate drug. Substances may even make your psychiatric symptoms better temporarily. After all, how can something that feels good or gets rid of symptoms be a problem?

Many addicted people have blackouts, or memory lapses. They forget things they've said or done while under the influence of alcohol or other drugs. Blackouts can prevent you from recognizing your addiction.

Another factor contributing to denial is the belief that you "always" have to lose control of alcohol or drug use to have a problem. Addiction is characterized by "inconsistent control," not total loss of control in all instances. Every alcoholic doesn't get drunk every time that he drinks. Every drug addict doesn't get high each time he uses drugs.

Euphoric recall can fuel the process of denial as well. This refers to remembering only the "positive" aspects of use. You may only remember the feelings of being high, buzzed up, mellow, or euphoric. Or, you may only remember "having fun or a good time" even though in reality you made a fool out of yourself, and embarrassed or upset other people.

Symptoms of many psychiatric illnesses are lack of insight and poor judgment. As a result of having an illness, you may deny that you are sick. For example, people who experience manic or psychotic episodes may not realize they are sick or are showing behaviors that threaten their safety or the safety of others. People with depression may deny their mood disorder by telling themselves everyone gets a bad case of the blues once in a while and that they need to pull themselves out of it. And, people with certain personality disorders blame all of their behaviors or problems on other people, bad breaks or bad luck, or society.

Recovery Activity

1. List an example of how you denied your psychiatric problem. *Example: "I told myself my depression wasn't bad enough to require treatment."*

    _____

    _____

    _____

2. List an example of how your denial of your addiction showed. *Example: "I thought that since pills and booze settled my nerves, how could these be a problem?"*

    _____

    _____

    _____

3. List an example of how others denied your disorder(s). *Example: "My husband got high with me. He told me all I needed was to cut down and control my drug use better, that I didn't need to stop completely."*

    _____

    _____

    _____

4. If you continue using alcohol or drugs, how will this affect your psychiatric condition? *Example: "It can make me stop taking my medications and relapse. I can end up back in the hospital."*

    _____

    _____

    _____

5. If you don't get help with your psychiatric disorder, how can this affect your addiction? *Example: "It'll be harder to stop using."*

    _____

    _____

    _____

13. Roadblocks to Recovery

There are many roadblocks or barriers that may interfere with your recovery.[1-3] You may resist recovery for different reasons. Admitting to a psychiatric problem can be hard. Giving up alcohol and other drugs, and changing yourself or your lifestyle can also be difficult. Recovery requires hard work on your part over a long period of time because there are no quick fixes or no easy ways to deal with co-occurring disorders.

Recovery barriers may relate to your attitudes, beliefs, feelings and motivation about recovery, your personality traits, your relationships with others, or your lifestyle. Being aware of these puts you in a position to do something about them.

1. I identify with these roadblocks related to my **attitudes or motivation.**
   - ❏ It's hard to admit I have a psychiatric disorder or need professional help.
   - ❏ It's hard to admit I have an alcohol or drug problem and need help.
   - ❏ I'm worried I can't stay off alcohol or other drugs.
   - ❏ I don't care about recovery.
   - ❏ I don't feel very capable or motivated to change.
   - ❏ My motivation changes day-to-day.
   - ❏ I'm only in treatment because of others and I don't want it for myself.
   - ❏ I'm angry at being in treatment.
   - ❏ I don't think the staff can help me or understand me.
   - ❏ I don't trust the staff (doctor, therapist, case manager, etc.).

2. I identify with these roadblocks related to my **participation in mutual support programs.**
   - ❏ I don't stick with AA, NA, dual recovery, or mental health support groups.
   - ❏ I don't have a sponsor or use the Twelve-Step program.
   - ❏ It's hard for me to talk about my "real" problems.
   - ❏ I don't follow through with treatment after I leave the hospital.
   - ❏ I don't like taking medications or don't take them as prescribed.
   - ❏ I miss too many partial hospital or outpatient sessions.
   - ❏ When I miss sessions, I don't reschedule them.
   - ❏ I quit treatment before I should.
   - ❏ I don't complete my therapy assignments.

3. I identify with these roadblocks relating to my **behaviors or personality.**
   - ❏ I don't want others telling me what to do.
   - ❏ I'm stubborn and have to do things my own way.
   - ❏ It's hard for me to change.
   - ❏ I'm too impulsive and often act before I think.
   - ❏ I'm too perfectionistic.
   - ❏ I give up too easily.

❑ I depend too much on others to figure out what to do.

❑ I use anger or hostility to keep people from getting to know me.

❑ I don't open up with others and keep my problems to myself.

4. I identify with these roadblocks in my **relationships.**

❑ I make suicidal threats or gestures when I don't get what I want, or am angry at others.

❑ My partner, spouse, or roommate gets high.

❑ I live with other family members or friends who get high.

❑ Most or all of my friends get high.

❑ It's hard for me to relate to people who don't get high.

❑ I don't have anyone I can lean on for support.

❑ It's hard for me to ask others for help.

❑ It's hard for me to trust other people.

❑ I don't feel close to anyone or loved by anyone.

❑ I don't like to listen to authority figures.

5. I identify with these roadblocks related to my **lifestyle.**

❑ My lifestyle centers on getting or using substances.

❑ I don't have any routine or structure in my life.

❑ My living situation is a threat to my recovery.

❑ I have little or no direction in my life.

❑ I have too much free time on my hands.

❑ I live mainly day-to-day without planning much for the future.

❑ I like hanging with a fast crowd, even if I'm not using.

❑ My life is a drag, and I don't have much to do that is rewarding or fun.

6. Other roadblocks are: _____

_____

_____

7. Identify two personal roadblocks to recovery and ways I can overcome each roadblock.

Roadblock 1 = _____

_____

Ways to overcome this roadblock to my recovery are: _____

_____

_____

_____

_____

Roadblock 2 = _____

_____

Ways to overcome this roadblock to my recovery are: _____

_____

_____

_____

_____

Example #1: Stan's Roadblocks and Plan

"I have a lot of roadblocks messing with my recovery. I'm tired of going in and out of rehabs, jails, and psychiatric hospitals. Been in too many times to count. Deep down, I'm scared I can't stay clean. But, man, the biggest obstacle to my recovery is me. I copped a bad attitude about treatment and other people telling me what to do to stop getting high and messing up my life. In treatment, I talk some good shit like I know what's going down. But ain't nothing gonna get better unless I do what they say in NA—quit talking the talk and walk the walk.

So here's what I want to do: get a sponsor and use him, go to meetings every day, and keep my mouth shut and listen to find out what recovery's all about. I'm going to keep all of my counseling sessions and stop bullshitting about why I shouldn't go. It ain't that hard, just be responsible and don't do things my way. My way just don't work, so it's time to try another way."

Example #2: Marissa's Roadblocks and Plan

"My two biggest roadblocks are stopping medications when my depression is better and not sticking with AA after I'm sober for a while. Even though I have recurrent depression and know I need ongoing medication, I sometimes stop after I feel good for several months. I do the same with AA. I'll be sober for months or a year or more, then convince myself I don't need AA.

My plan is simple. I've made an agreement with my doctor and therapist that I will talk with them whenever I start thinking I can stop my medication. And, I'll review my list of the reasons I need to continue antidepressants even when my mood has been stable for months or longer. I'll do the same with AA meetings by talking with my sponsor or therapist to review the purpose and benefits of AA *before* I privately decide to reduce frequency or stop meetings completely. I'll also remind myself that both my depression and alcoholism are chronic, lifelong diseases, and recovery is ongoing even if it is day by day."

14. Recovery from Co-Occurring Disorders

Recovery from co-occurring disorders involves addressing your psychiatric illness, your addiction, and the problems contributing to or resulting from your disorders.[1] Recovery is a *long-term process* that requires effort on your part and a willingness to get actively involved in improving yourself. It involves:

- Getting sober from alcohol or drugs
- Stabilizing from acute psychiatric symptoms
- Learning about your illnesses, treatment and recovery
- Motivating yourself to change because you want to get well
- Developing realistic attitudes about recovery and change
- Learning and using skills to stay sober from alcohol or drugs
- Learning and using skills to manage your psychiatric disorder
- Actively working a recovery program that focuses on your co-occurring disorders and making positive changes in yourself and your lifestyle
- Developing a plan to reduce relapse risk and deal with emergencies

Phases of Recovery

There are different phases of recovery that you may go through.[2] Each phase has issues that are common to people in recovery. However, not every person progresses through these phases in the same way or at the same rate. Keep this in mind as you read about these phases of recovery. Factors determining your progression include the severity of your disorders, your personality, your coping style, your support network, and your motivation to work a recovery program.

Transition and Engagement

This phase involves becoming engaged in treatment, either voluntarily or as a result of an involuntary commitment. This involves some recognition that you haven't been able to control your use of alcohol or other drugs, or that your psychiatric disorder requires treatment. However, in cases of involuntary commitment involving severe psychiatric symptoms, recognition may not occur until there is some stability of your acute symptoms.

Your alcohol or drug use may have played a major role in a new episode of psychiatric illness following a period of remission. Or, your substance use may have led to a worsening of existing psychiatric symptoms such as depression, mania, psychosis, suicidality, anxiety, panic, out of control or threatening behaviors toward others, or an inability to function and take care of your basic needs. In some cases, your alcohol or drug use may have "masked" your psychiatric symptoms, prolonging your entry into treatment.

During this phase, you begin to recognize that an untreated psychiatric disorder interferes with your ability to remain sober from alcohol or other drugs or negatively affects your motivation and desire to recover from addiction. You may engage in treatment in a psychiatric hospital or outpatient setting, or an addiction rehabilitation setting, depending on the nature and severity of your symptoms. If you enter treatment through a psychiatric system, you may eventually be referred to an addiction rehabilitation program if this is essential for you to initiate recovery from addiction.

In this phase, you begin to come to grips with your mixed feelings about recovery, accepting the reality that part of you wants to stop using substances and get well and part of you doesn't want to stop using substances or make any changes. The same holds true for your psychiatric illness—you begin to accept that part of you that needs help and part of you doesn't think you need any help and that you can get well on your own.

If possible, your family should get involved in your treatment. They can provide helpful information to professionals who care for you, emotional support to you, and they can gain much from treatment for themselves. The earlier they get involved in the assessment and treatment processes, the better it usually is for everyone involved.

You also begin to accept the need for a recovery program that involves a combination of professional treatment and mutual support programs such as AA, NA, Cocaine Anonymous (CA), Dual Recovery Anonymous (DRA), or other mental health support groups. You learn that you need help and support from others to recover from your disorders. Your motivation to change at first may be "external" as you get involved mainly because of the problems your addiction and mental health disorder have caused, or because you have been "forced" or "pressured" to accept help by your family, employer, the court system, a health care or social service professional, or some other important person in your life.

This phase may take several weeks or longer, although for some it takes months or years to become truly engaged in dual diagnosis recovery and motivated to change. Some enter treatment only to drop out early. If you make a commitment to stay in recovery, even if you feel your motivation is questionable, you put yourself in a good position to benefit from treatment. Keep in mind that many people need time to develop motivation to recover, and that staying in treatment "buys you time" to develop this motivation and see the many potential benefits of treatment.

Stabilization

This phase involves stabilizing your acute psychiatric symptoms. You may receive medications to help stabilize your symptoms. Depending on the nature of your symptoms and your past response to medications, it may take several weeks or longer for medications to reduce or eliminate your symptoms. This requires patience on your part and a willingness to stick with treatment even if you feel frustrated. In some cases, stabilizing from an episode of psychiatric illness is a smooth process. In other cases, it is much more complex and takes longer.

This recovery phase also involves getting alcohol and drugs out of your system and adjusting to being substance-free. For some people, medical detoxification is needed to break the cycle of addiction. Acute symptoms of withdrawal from alcohol or other drugs usually last a few days to a week or so. The specific withdrawal symptoms depend on the amount and types of substances you have been using. Protracted or post-acute withdrawal symptoms may last for weeks or months. If your body adapted to heavy use of alcohol or other drugs for years, you can't expect it to adjust to being substance-free in just a few short days.

Learn about your illnesses (diagnoses, symptoms, causes, effects), the role of therapy, medications and mutual support programs in ongoing recovery. Knowledge empowers you and helps you know what you can do to help yourself. In this phase of recovery you can learn ways to cope with addictive thinking, cravings to use alcohol or drugs and symptoms of your psychiatric illness. Get involved in mutual support programs such as AA, NA, or CA for your addiction; Double Trouble in Recovery (DTR), mentally ill substance abuser (MISA), substance abusing mentally ill (SAMI), chemical abusing mentally ill (CAMI), or DRA programs for your co-occurring disorders; or mental health support groups based on the nature of your psychiatric illness (for example, anxiety disorder support groups or manic-depression support groups).

As you progress through this phase of recovery, you become less preoccupied with alcohol and other drugs. You learn to counteract euphoric recall and positive thoughts about using substances to reduce your risk of relapsing. Your motivation gets stronger as you learn that there are many steps you can take to help your recovery. And, you become more comfortable accepting help and support from others so you don't recover alone.

Accept the need for long-term involvement in recovery. Work closely with your treatment team to develop a list of problems to work on, prioritize these and develop strategies to address select problems from your list. Accepting the need for total abstinence from alcohol, street drugs, and non-prescribed drugs puts you in a position to get the most from your recovery.

Your family's involvement should continue in this phase as well. The degree to which they are involved and the nature of their involvement depends on your needs, their needs, and the recommendations of the professionals providing treatment to you.

This phase of recovery may take weeks or up to several months or even longer. The ease with which you move through this stage depends on the severity of your psychiatric illness and your addiction, as well as the type of treatment you are receiving.

Early Recovery

This phase of recovery involves continued work at recovery from both of your disorders. You stay sober by coping with cravings and desires to use substances, avoiding high-risk people, places, and things that represent a relapse risk for you. Since you cannot avoid all risk factors, you use active coping strategies to resist pressures from others to use alcohol or other drugs. You become more used to sobriety and coping with the many adjustments that it brings. During this phase, you begin to make internal changes by learning how to combat your addictive thinking. Your "sober" side takes a stronger role than your "addicted" side and you more openly embrace the need for a recovery program that accepts total abstinence as the best goal for you. You still want to use at times, but you know this is part of an addictive disease and that you can cope with this part if you use the tools of the program that you have been learning.

During early recovery, you learn ways to cope with your psychiatric disorder and the problems it caused. While medication can help improve symptoms of your illness, you have to work at making changes in yourself and your lifestyle in order to promote a better recovery. You learn to challenge and change negative thinking that contributed to anxiety, depression or unhappiness. You become more realistic about recovery and the need for active involvement in a program of change.

Early recovery also involves building structure and regularity into your day-to-day life so that you keep busy, stay focused on recovery issues, get involved in leisure activities that are enjoyable, and don't have a lot of free time on your hands. Structure helps you stay focused on your goals and can serve as a protective factor against relapse to your disorders.

In family sessions, focus on understanding the impact of your disorders and behaviors on your family. Learn how your family can support your recovery and how you can support them. You and your family may need to learn to communicate more openly about recovery. This helps set the stage for making amends later.

Involvement in therapy and mutual support programs helps you with these issues. Working the Twelve Steps becomes an important aspect of your change plan, as does working with a sponsor who can guide you in using the "tools" of recovery.

As you progress through this stage, you feel less guilty and shameful because you learn that you are not a "bad person," but that your disorders contributed to unhealthy behaviors. You accept responsibility for coping with your disorders by staying involved in treatment and mutual support programs.

Early recovery roughly involves three to six months after the stabilization phase. Similar to previous phases, some work through this phase more easily than others. If you relapse to alcohol or drug use, or experience a worsening of your psychiatric symptoms, you will need to stabilize before you can address many of the issues discussed on the previous page.

Middle Recovery

This phase builds on work from early recovery. In therapy, you share more about your inner thoughts and feelings and reach a greater level of self-awareness. You work on improving your relationships by communicating more openly with others. You become more caring and loving toward others. You not only "get" support and help from others, but you also "give" to others, too. This helps you develop more balanced relationships.

In middle recovery, you spend more time and effort repairing the damage to your relationships and self-esteem caused by your disorders. Steps 8 and 9 of AA, NA, CA, or DRA are addressed with your sponsor and/or therapist. These steps help you identify others hurt by your behaviors, become willing to make amends and figure out ways to make amends when doing so will not bring harm to other people. Your relationships become more meaningful and satisfying as a result. In relationships where damage can't be repaired and the relationships can't be salvaged, you learn to accept this reality rather than judge yourself harshly.

Spirituality issues in recovery become more important during this phase. You further develop your own unique sense of spirituality and use this to help your recovery and growth as a person. This process may or may not also involve active participation in some formal type of religion. As you progress through this phase of recovery, you focus more on becoming a better person and being satisfied with yourself. Steps 10 and 11 can help in this process.

You continue improving how you cope with negative or upsetting thoughts and feelings. You change anxious, depressed or other negative thinking patterns. You realize that by changing your thinking, you can change your feelings as well as how you act. As you make changes in different areas of yourself and your life, your self-esteem rises. You feel less demoralized and victimized by your disorders. Instead, you see the need to continue making changes in yourself. You stop blaming society, bad breaks, bad genes, or others for your problems.

Since addictive and psychiatric disorders are often chronic, relapsing illnesses, you learn to identify and manage warning signs of relapse. You learn that going back to using alcohol and drugs doesn't usually "come out of the blue," but represents a movement away from recovery toward relapse over time. Similarly, you learn that new episodes of psychiatric illness or significant worsening of persistent and chronic psychiatric symptoms often occur gradually. Knowing your potential relapse warning signs allows you to develop strategies that reduce the likelihood of relapse to either or both of your disorders. Your relapse-prevention plan becomes an important part of recovery. By monitoring your recovery on a daily basis, you put yourself in a position to spot relapse warning signs early. This allows you to take action before things get out of hand.

If your psychiatric illness was a first episode and you are fairly free of symptoms as a result of treatment, you may be withdrawn from medications. Usually, this is not done until you have been doing well for four months or longer. If you have a recurrent psychiatric disorder or a chronic, persistent form of illness such as schizophrenia, bipolar illness or recurrent major depression, you likely will remain on medications even if you are doing well. The purpose of medications is to "prevent" a recurrence of psychiatric illness. The idea is similar to taking medications for high blood pressure or other medical illnesses—taking medicine maintains treatment gains and helps prevent future symptoms. It is still possible for symptoms to break through even if you take medications. However, this happens less often than in cases when medications are stopped prematurely.

Middle recovery usually involves the six to twelve month period following early recovery. As in other phases, some move through this phase more easily than others.

Late Recovery

This phase of recovery involves continued work started in the previous phases. Usually, you get into personal recovery issues in greater depth after you have established a solid foundation for your recovery. You focus more on changing your "character defects" and dealing with other problems caused by your personality style. You build on your strengths and work on your weaknesses.

You may also work at finding greater meaning in life and developing more positive values. The spiritual and interpersonal aspects of recovery help you in this quest. One of the benefits of recovery is that it provides you a chance to become a better, more fulfilled person. But this only comes with patience, discipline, and hard work.

If you are in therapy, focus may shift away from practical daily life issues and more toward greater self-exploration so that you better understand yourself—your defenses, your personality style, your patterns of behavior, your values and your strengths. You gain greater clarity on how your past influences you at the present time. Greater self-understanding helps pave the way to make personal changes and improve yourself.

As you progress through this phase, you become more able and willing to focus on healing from past emotional wounds related to growing up in a family where a serious addiction or mental health problem existed, or related to other traumatic experiences. You face your pain head-on rather than use it as a reason to drink alcohol or use drugs, or as a reason not to change your life. Gradually, you let go of your anger, disappointment, and sadness. And, you learn to forgive others whom you feel harmed you in the past. If you are unable or unwilling to forgive, you learn to live with your pain and anger in ways that aren't self-destructive.

In some instances this healing takes place by working the Twelve-Step program of AA, NA, CA, or DRA. In other cases, it involves deeper exploration in therapy sessions. Therapy helps you slowly work through your pain and put it in a different perspective so that it doesn't continue to cause you so much emotional pain. To aid your healing journey, you may also participate in other types of self-help support groups such as Adult Children of Alcoholics (ACA), Incest Survivors Anonymous, or codependency groups.

Late recovery also gives you the opportunity to work at "balancing" the various areas of your life—recovery, work, love, relationships, fun, and spirituality. This phase lasts roughly one to two years after the middle recovery period.

Maintenance

This final phase is best seen as an "ongoing" phase. It involves continued work on your "self" in recovery. You shift toward more self-reliance during this phase and rely less on others for help. You still need and depend on others, but you rely more and more on your own inner resources to cope with your thoughts, feelings, and problems in life.

Part of your continued growth and development may come from "giving away" what you learned in recovery by sponsoring others and working Step 12. You are able to use your experience, hope, and strength to help others in recovery.

Since you are well-grounded in recovery by this time, you are better able to deal with the problems life brings you on a daily basis. You face these head-on, whatever they are. Coping with problems and changes in your life doesn't overwhelm you like it did in the early phases of recovery.

You learn to cope with setbacks and mistakes that you make in your life and recovery. You use your mistakes to learn something new about yourself or life rather than as a reason to put yourself down. You become more accepting of your limitations, weaknesses, and flaws. You modify your goals in life if you discover you can't reach them or that they were set too high in the first place.

During the maintenance phase, if you have a recurrent or persistent form of psychiatric illness, you continue taking medications. By this phase, you will have decreased the frequency in which you see a therapist or psychiatrist as you are busy "living the program" of recovery.

As the name of this phase implies, it is ongoing. You "maintain" gains made previously while continuing to grow as a person.

If you have a setback and relapse to your addiction or psychiatric illness, you won't necessarily have to go through all of these phases again. This all depends on the nature of your relapse, how long it lasts, and the damage it does to you and your relationships.

Try to avoid comparing yourself to others because everyone works differently in recovery. Measure your progress in relation to previous periods of illness. Even if you are still having problems, it is possible that you are still making progress and moving in the right direction. Remember, progress sometimes comes in small steps.

Areas of Recovery

A way to look at your recovery plan is to think about the different areas of your life, and identify changes you want to make. Your recovery plan may involve any of the following areas:

Physical

Getting regular physical, dental and eye exams, ensuring that you get enough sleep and rest, eating nutritious meals and eating regularly, exercising to keep in shape and release built-up tension, learning how to relax and deal with stress, dealing with cravings or strong desires to use alcohol or drugs and following your treatment plan if you are being treated for any type of medical problem.

Emotional

Working through denial and accepting both of your disorders and the need to change, developing skills to cope with your feelings, thoughts, and problems, working through emotional wounds from the past, improving your self-esteem, and coping with persistent symptoms of your psychiatric illness.

Family and interpersonal

Evaluating the impact of your disorders and behaviors on your family and other people, making amends when appropriate, building a recovery-support system and healthy relationships, encouraging your family to get involved in treatment sessions with you and/or mutual support groups for families (e.g., Al-Anon, Nar-Anon, Families of the Mentally Ill), improving your communication skills, and improving the quality of your relationships.

Social and leisure

Spending time in social and leisure activities that bring you enjoyment and satisfaction, making sure you don't isolate yourself from other people, avoiding people, places, and things associated with getting drunk or high, learning how to say no when other people offer you alcohol or drugs, and learning how to have fun without needing alcohol or drugs.

Lifestyle

Building structure and routine into your daily life so you keep busy and are engaged in constructive work, leisure, social, or recovery activities; learning how to manage money; setting goals that you want to work toward achieving; and dealing with any legal, financial, job, school, or other problems.

Spiritual

Developing your faith, spiritual or religious beliefs, finding meaning in your life, becoming active in your religion, relying on God or your Higher Power for inner strength, praying or reading the Bible or other spiritual materials.

Daily inventory

Monitoring your progress on a daily basis to keep track of your symptoms and problems to determine if you are getting better or sliding backwards. A daily inventory helps you catch relapse warning signs and problems early so you can face them head-on rather than wait until things build up too much.

Recovery Activity

1. Which phase of recovery do you think you are in? Explain your answer.

   _____

   _____

   _____

   _____

   _____

   _____

2. Of the areas of recovery discussed, list two that are most important to you at this time. Then, for each one, list steps you can take to work on each recovery issue.

   Recovery Issue #1 _____

   _____

   Steps to take: _____

   _____

   _____

   _____

   _____

   Recovery Issue #2 _____

   _____

   Steps to take: _____

15. Coping with Cravings for Alcohol or Drugs

Cravings for alcohol or other drugs are common when you first stop using.[1] One craving may be so strong and intense that you feel like you'll go crazy if you don't use. Another craving may be no big deal. Your cravings may be "overt" which means that you know you are craving alcohol or drugs. Or, your cravings may be "covert," which means you don't know you want alcohol or drugs. For example, some people become very irritable, upset and edgy when they first enter a hospital or rehabilitation program. They become critical of staff, other patients and recovery. Some even check themselves out against medical advice. In many cases, what lies beneath the surface and is a major reason for this irritability or edginess is a hidden craving for alcohol or drugs.

Cravings are triggered by many different *internal factors* such as feeling anxious, angry, or edgy. *External factors* that trigger cravings include people, places, events, things or objects, rituals or experiences that remind you of using or being high. Sometimes, you don't need anything to trigger it. Your addiction itself can cause cravings.

It helps to know the common triggers that cause alcohol or drug cravings. It also helps to figure out your own craving triggers. Once you know your triggers and how your cravings show, you can then develop coping strategies to help you cope with a craving so you don't use chemicals. The following exercise shows you one way to understand your alcohol and drug cravings.

1. My internal craving triggers are:

   • Feelings _____

   _____

   • Thoughts _____

   _____

   • Physical sensations or symptoms_____

   _____

2. Factors in my environment (external triggers) that cause cravings to get high are:

   • People (for example, other users, spouse or partner, the dealer) _____

   _____

   • Places (e.g., bars, clubs, a specific house, building or room, car, neighborhood) _____

   _____

   • Events associated with using (e.g., parties, sporting events, concerts, payday, check day)

   _____

   _____

- Things or objects associated with using or preparing substances (e.g., seeing or smelling alcohol or drugs, needles, coke spoons, pipes and bongs, papers, music, money)

  _____

  _____

  _____

- Other situations (e.g., getting a flu shot, visiting a doctor) _____

  _____

  _____

3. Do you have drugs or paraphernalia (pipes, needles, etc.) in your home? ❑ yes ❑ no
   If yes, why and what are you going to do with them? _____

   _____

   _____

4. Do you keep alcohol in your home? ❑ yes ❑ no
   If yes, why and how can this affect your recovery? _____

   _____

   _____

5. Positive ways to help me resist the desire to use when I crave alcohol or drugs are: _____

   _____

   _____

6. If I am able to cope successfully with cravings I will feel: _____

   _____

   _____

7. If I give in to my cravings I will feel: _____

   _____

   _____

Managing Your Cravings

1. **Recognize and label your craving.** Know the signs of your cravings and the triggers. Use whatever label is comfortable for you: craving, desire, urge, or drug or alcohol hunger.
2. **Talk about your craving.** Talk with your sponsor, an AA, NA, CA or other friend, counselor, or family member. This may provide relief and you may hear how others coped with cravings. Talking may increase your craving at first. If this happens, use other coping strategies.
3. **Go to a mutual support group meeting (e.g., AA, NA, CA).** This can provide you with support. You can discuss your craving with others and hear how they have coped with theirs.

4. **Use self-talk.** Tell yourself you won't use, or that you'll put off using for a few hours or days. By that time, your craving will pass. Think positive and tell yourself you'll get through your craving. Remind yourself of the benefits of not using and problems if you use again. Imagine that you can talk to your craving and tell it to "go to hell" and that you won't let it defeat you. Remind yourself that the more struggles with cravings that you win, the stronger you will feel.

5. **Accept that it will pass.** Sometimes all you need to do is accept the fact that cravings will come and go. You don't have to use just because you have a craving. Remember, it will pass.

6. **Do something active—now!** This can help redirect your energies and divert your attention. Make a list of activities that you can keep busy with if your craving gets strong. Hobbies, sports, or other physical activities can help you cope with your cravings.

7. **Write in a journal.** Put your thoughts and feelings into words and write them in a journal. Describe your cravings and the situations in which they occur. Keep track of the outcome of your craving and positive coping strategies you used. Keeping a regular journal may even help you figure out if there are patterns to your cravings.

8. **Get rid of booze, drugs and paraphernalia.** Don't keep alcohol and drugs in your home. Get rid of drug paraphernalia such as papers, pipes, needles, and mirrors.

9. **Keep a craving coping card in your wallet or purse.** Write down a list of positive coping strategies and carry on a 3 x 5 index card in your wallet or purse. Review this to remind yourself of positive strategies to deal with cravings.

10. **Be aware of high-risk people, places, and situations.** There may be people, places, or situations that you must avoid to not put yourself at risk to use, especially during times when you feel a strong craving. Since you can't avoid all high-risk people or situations, be prepared ahead of time so that you can cope with cravings or desires to use if they pop up.

11. **Pray.** Ask God or your Higher Power for help and strength to get through your craving. Use your faith and religious beliefs or practices.

12. **Read recovery literature.** Read passages from the AA *Big Book*, the NA *Basic Text*, or other books and guides on recovery. Reading may provide you with coping strategies, inspire you to continue your recovery journey, or calm you down.

Example: Carol's Triggers and Plan

"I have lots of triggers. The ones I'm dealing with now are feeling pissed off or upset or being around people I got high with. When I'm mad or upset, I'll pick up the phone instead of a drug. I'll call my sponsor or NA friends. I'll work hard to fight off desires to get high by telling my craving to go to hell that I will control it, it won't control me and I ain't going to use under any circumstance. I got rid of booze and drugs in my house and I'm not going to hang with people who get high. I'll start each day with a reminder of why I want to stay sober today and what I'm grateful for in my recovery."

SECTION IV

Managing Emotions

16. Managing Anger

Anger problems are common among people with co-occurring disorders.[1,2] Friction can be caused in a relationship if you ignore your anger or act on it in ways that hurt others physically or emotionally. Anger problems can interfere with recovery if you don't cope with these feelings in positive ways.

Anger can also empower you if dealt with in a positive way. It can motivate you to set or reach goals or work hard to accomplish things in your life.

It is not your feelings of anger that causes problems but how you think about and express it that determines how anger affects your life. Some people try to ignore their anger and let it build up. They stew on the inside and become upset or depressed. They express anger indirectly by dragging their feet, forgetting dates that are important to people they feel anger toward, criticizing others behind their backs, or avoiding people they are mad at.

Other people let their anger out much too quickly and impulsively. They lash out at others and yell, cuss, scream, or act in other hostile ways. Some become violent, get into fights, or destroy objects or property. Violence is a significant problem for some people with a substance abuse or psychiatric disorder.[3]

Recovery Activity

1. How much of a problem is your anger or how you cope with it?
    ❑ No problem ❑ Small problem ❑ Moderate problem ❑ Serious problem

2. My anger usually shows in these ways (e.g., I get sad, frustrated, pace, feel nervous):

    _____

    _____

    _____

3. I usually deal with anger by (e.g., holding it inside, letting it out immediately, talking it out, lashing out at others, fighting):

    _____

    _____

    _____

4. My anger affects my physical or mental health in the following ways:

    _____

    _____

5. My anger affects my relationships in the following ways:

    _____

    _____

6. My anger affects my use of alcohol or other drugs by:

    _____

    _____

7. I can use my anger in a positive way by:

    _____

    _____

Strategies for Managing Anger

1. **Recognize angry feelings.** Pay attention to body cues, thoughts, and behaviors that tell you that you are angry. Use cues to admit you are angry. Don't deny, hide, minimize, or ignore it.

2. **Figure out why you are angry.** When you feel angry figure out of where it is coming from. Does it relate to something another person did or said to you? Does it relate to an event, experience, or situation? Or, is your anger caused by the way you think about things?

3. **Decide if you should feel angry.** Are you an angry person who seems to get mad too often or for no good reason? When angry, ask yourself if the facts of the situation warrant an angry reaction on your part. Or, ask yourself if your anger is the result of a character defect (i.e., you get mad frequently for little things).

4. **Identify the effects of your anger and your methods of coping with anger.** How does your anger and your methods of coping with it affect your physical, mental, or spiritual health? How are your relationships with family members, friends, or others affected?

5. **Use different strategies to deal with anger.** These include cognitive (your beliefs about anger and the internal messages you give yourself), behavioral (how you act), and verbal (what you say to other people) strategies. Having a variety of strategies puts you in a good position to cope with anger in a wide range of situations.

6. **Use cognitive strategies for anger management such as:**
    *   Evaluating your beliefs about anger and changing those that cause you problems. If you believe you should "let it out" every time you get angry, you may find this isn't always the best policy and that this belief should be modified. Or, if you believe you should never get mad, you might have to change this belief and give yourself permission to feel anger.
    *   Catching yourself when you are angry and changing your angry thoughts. Determine if your anger is justified given the situation. This requires not jumping to conclusions and examining all of the facts of the situation first.
    *   Using positive self-talk or slogans (for example, "this too will pass," "keep your cool and stay in control").
    *   Using fantasy. Imagine yourself coping in a positive way.
    *   Evaluating the risks and benefits of expressing your anger or holding it inside.
    *   Reminding yourself of negative effects of ignoring anger and holding it inside.
    *   Reminding yourself of negative effects of expressing anger in hurtful ways.
    *   Identifying the benefits of handling anger in a positive way.

- Taking a few minutes at the end of the day to see if you are harboring any anger from the events of the day.

7. **Use verbal strategies for anger management such as:**
   - Sharing your feelings with whom you are angry. Discuss the situation or problem that contributed to your anger.
   - Sharing your angry feelings with a friend, family member, therapist or sponsor. Many find it helpful to discuss anger at support group meetings.
   - Discussing the situation or problem that contributed to your anger with a neutral person to get their opinion on the situation.
   - Apologizing or making amends to others who were hurt as a result of how you expressed your anger.

8. **Use behavior strategies for anger management such as:**
   - Directing anger toward physical activity such as walking, exercise, or sports.
   - Directing feelings of anger toward some type of work.
   - Expressing self with painting, drawing, and other forms of arts and crafts.
   - Writing about your feelings in a journal or anger log.
   - Practicing verbal strategies mentioned in the previous section so you feel better prepared to express your feelings to others.
   - Using reminder cards that provide you with specific coping strategies you can use to deal with anger.
   - Leaving situations when your anger is so intense you worry about losing control and doing something irrational or violent.

Seek professional help if you experience serious problems as a result of anger and how you cope with it, or are unable to gain better control of it on your own. Professional help is especially important for those who act out angry impulses by hitting or hurting others or breaking objects. Professional treatment also can help those who turn anger against themselves and exhibit self-destructive tendencies such as those who cut, burn, or hurt themselves.

17. *Managing Anxiety and Worry*

Most people feel anxious and worry at times. However, some people experience excessive anxiety and worry so much that it causes a lot of distress. Anxiety symptoms are common among people with addiction, depression, or other psychiatric disorders.[1,2] Many use alcohol or drugs to decrease anxiety only to find in the long run such use leads to alcohol or drug problems or, they avoid situations that cause their anxious feelings. Anxiety is quite common when a person first stops drinking alcohol or using drugs. It is a common withdrawal symptom and has both a physical and psychological basis.

Anxiety refers to the physical side and worry refers to the mental side. When you have one, you usually have the other. Anxiety shows in physical symptoms such as: shortness of breath, rapid heartbeat, tightness or discomfort in the chest, feeling lightheaded or weak, feeling uptight or on edge, or tingling and numbness.

Anticipatory anxiety refers to feeling anxious when you think ahead of time what "may happen" at some event or situation in the future. Some people avoid situations because of this. Some situations they may avoid include: shopping, standing in check-out lines in stores, writing in public, attending church, going to the doctor or dentist, going to movies, sporting events or music concerts, driving through tunnels or over bridges, riding elevators or escalators, or traveling by plane, bus or train. Some people become so anxious and fearful of leaving home that they seldom or never leave their home. When they do leave home, they often need another person to go along with them.

Worry refers to thinking about things over and over in your head in relation to a *real* problem or a *potential* problem (something you think might happen). People who worry a lot may believe that they cannot cope with the problems or situations they worry about.

Recovery Activities

1. How much of a problem is your anxiety or how you cope with it?
   ❑ No problem   ❑ Small problem   ❑ Moderate problem   ❑ Serious problem

2. How much of a problem is your worry or how you cope with it?
   ❑ No problem   ❑ Small problem   ❑ Moderate problem   ❑ Serious problem

3. My anxiety shows in the following ways: _____

   _____

   _____

4. The reasons I get anxious are: _____

   _____

   _____

5. My anxiety and worry have affected my life in the following ways:

   _____

   _____

   _____

6.   My anxiety and worry have affected my relationships in the following ways: _____

_____

_____

7.   I worry a lot about these situations or events: _____

_____

_____

8.   The connection between my use of alcohol or drugs and my anxiety or worry is:

_____

_____

_____

Strategies for Managing Anxiety and Worry

1.   **Identify and label anxiety and worry.** Know the signs and symptoms of excessive anxiety or worry. This will help you "catch" yourself when you feel anxious or are worrying too much.

2.   **Find out what is causing your anxiety and worry.** Identify the specific problems, situations, or things that cause you to feel anxious and worried. If these are real problems, look at ways to solve these. If these are *potential* problems, ask yourself if these problems will really occur. Work on changing how you think about potential problems.

3.   **Get a physical examination.** This can help determine if medical problems are contributing to your anxiety.

4.   **Evaluate your diet.** Take a close look at what you are eating or taking into your body. Try to figure out if your use of caffeine, sugar, or other foods is contributing to anxiety and making you feel on edge.

5.   **Evaluate your lifestyle.** Make sure you are getting enough rest, relaxation, and exercise. Exercise can help release some of your anxious feelings. It may serve the additional benefit of helping prevent anxious feelings from building up. Meditation and relaxation techniques can also help reduce your anxiety.

6.   **Use proper breathing techniques.** Stop shallow or rapid breathing or holding your breath. Learn proper ways of breathing and practice these each day until they become automatic. You can practice breathing techniques anywhere—at work, home, in the car, before a speech, or before going into a situation when you feel anxious.

7.   **Change your beliefs or thoughts.** Practice changing your "anxious" and "worrisome" thoughts or beliefs. When working on a *real* problem causing your anxiety or worry, view the problem for what it is. Don't see it as a barrier that you can't overcome. When feeling real anxious or worried about a *potential* problem, ask yourself what evidence you have that the problem will ever occur or the outcome will be what you fear it will be. Try to identify all possible outcomes, not just the negative ones that you worry will happen. Make positive self-statements,

such as "I can do it," "My anxiety won't get the best of me," "I'm in control of my worry," "It's OK to make mistakes," or "No one has to be perfect."

8. **Share your anxious feelings and thoughts with others.** Discussing your feelings and worries with a friend, family member, sponsor, or counselor may help you feel better and gain relief. This can also help you learn what others do to handle their anxiety and worry and identify new ways to cope. However, keep in mind that you can overwhelm others if you constantly share your worries. If you share your feelings and don't make attempts at getting better, you might turn others off. People usually don't mind hearing their friend's or loved one's feelings unless the same old story is told over and over.

9. **Set aside "worry" time each day.** Try to avoid worrying throughout the day and save your worries for a time of the day that you call your "worry time." Pick a place and regular time and allow yourself to let your worries out. Don't go on endlessly and limit yourself to no more than one-half hour a day for this worry time.

10. **Keep a written anxiety and worry journal.** Writing your thoughts and feelings in a journal will help you release and better understand your thoughts and feelings. This can also help identify patterns to your anxiety and worry, coping strategies that don't work, and coping strategies that work in reducing anxiety and worry. This can also help track your progress over time.

11. **Face the situations causing you to feel anxious and worry.** Reality is often not as bad as what you think it will be. When you directly face the situations you find difficult, your confidence level should increase. Start with the least threatening anxiety or worry provoking situations and gradually build up toward facing the more difficult ones. Engaging in situations you feel anxious and worry about should reduce your anxiety and worry.

12. **If your anxiety continues to cause you significant distress, seek help from a mental health professional.** A mental health professional (e.g., psychiatrist, psychologist, social worker, or counselor) can help determine if your anxiety is a symptom of a psychiatric illness. Many types of treatment are available for anxiety disorders. These include different types of psychotherapy as well as medication. Be careful about types of medication used as it is easy to become dependent on medications such as tranquilizers. Let your doctor know that you are recovering from a alcohol or drug problem so proper medications are used should your symptoms be serious enough to require the use of medicine.

18. Coping with Boredom

Managing your boredom is an important part of recovery. Many people say feelings of boredom give them an excuse to drink alcohol or use other drugs. If your lifestyle was wrapped up in alcohol or drugs, or in the "fast life," being clean or sober may feel boring at first. You may miss the "action" associated with getting or using substances even more than you miss alcohol or drugs.

You need to replace drug and alcohol activities with new ones so boredom is not an excuse to use substances again. Perhaps, like many others, you gave up some of your non-drug and alcohol interests over time as your addiction took over your life.

You may also feel bored with your job, your relationships or other life circumstances. Substance use may have covered up your boredom. Figure out why you are bored with your life. For example, maybe you are bored in your primary relationship because your needs aren't being met. Or, maybe you are bored at work because you aren't able to use your talents or your job isn't challenging.

Answer the following questions to assess where you stand in relation to boredom and to see how your addiction may have contributed to it.

1. How much of a problem is your boredom or how you cope with it?
    ❑ No problem   ❑ Small problem   ❑ Moderate problem   ❑ Serious problem

2. I enjoy the following hobbies or activities:_____

    _____

    _____

3. As a result of my alcohol or drug problem I gave up these activities: _____

    _____

    _____

4. I would like to get involved in these activities again:_____

    _____

    _____

5. New activities or interests I would like to get involved in that do not involve a risk of using alcohol or other drugs include: _____

    _____

    _____

6. I am (or am not) bored and in need of a lot of "action" or excitement: _____

    _____

    _____

7. What excites me and makes me feel good about life is:_____

    _____

    _____

Strategies for Managing Boredom

1. **Regain lost activities.** Get involved in activities not associated with substance use that you enjoyed before your addiction took over your life.

2. **Develop new leisure interests.** Learn new hobbies, develop new interests, or find new forms of pleasure or enjoyment. Think of something you always wanted to do but never quite got around to doing, and try it. There really are endless activities or hobbies you could get involved in. Find those that interest you and do them!

3. **Build structure into your daily life.** The more structured your life is, the less time you have to feel bored. Build fun and relaxation into your day-to-day life so it isn't only focused on work, responsibilities or recovery. Find a balance in leisure activities involving other people, and those involving just yourself. While it is good to socialize with others and share mutual interests and activities, it is also good to have things to do that you can enjoy while you are alone.

4. **Know your high risk times for boredom.** Identify "high-risk" times for feeling bored and plan activities during these times. For most people in recovery, weekends and evenings are the toughest. Force yourself to get active in social activities.

5. **Participate in social activities sponsored by Twelve-Step groups or recovery clubs.** Many Twelve-Step programs sponsor social or recreational activities. Likewise, recovery clubs offer a sober atmosphere to relate to others and participate in social events such as dances or dinners.

6. **Think differently about boredom.** Change your attitudes and beliefs about boredom. Expect some boredom in your life. Even though it helps to structure your time, don't think you always have to be busy or engaged in fun. It's OK to have time for yourself that isn't planned.

7. **Focus on enjoying the simple things in life.** If you have a need for high levels of action, excitement or risk, learn to enjoy some of the simple pleasures in life. Don't expect to always be able to satisfy your need for "action" or excitement. Life simply doesn't work that way.

8. **Improve relationships and initiate activities with others.** Nurture and improve relationships and find new friends. Positive relationships add richness to your life, especially if you share mutual interests or activities with others. If you feel bored or lonely and want to be with others, take the initiative. Call others and invite them to share a mutual interest. Don't expect to always do what you want. Instead, learn to enjoy what others like to do. But make sure you spend time doing things that are fun and enjoyable to you.

9. **Go slow in making major life changes.** Carefully evaluate relationship or job boredom before making any major changes. Don't make quick or impulsive changes. Before you make any change, examine the potential risk and benefits. If you are bored with your spouse, partner or mate, figure out why and how to make things better before deciding to end the relationship.

10. **Use therapy to help with feelings of emptiness.** If you feel very empty inside and nothing seems to have meaning or purpose in your life, consult a professional mental health therapist. You may benefit from therapy. A severe feeling of emptiness sometimes is a symptom of a psychiatric illness such as depression or a personality problem.

19. *Managing Depression*

Many people with alcohol and drug problems experience depression.[1,2] Alcohol, opiates, tranquilizers, and sedatives depress the central nervous system and can cause you to feel depressed. Depression is also associated with "crashing" from the effects of cocaine or other stimulant drugs. Problems and losses caused by alcohol or drug use can cause feelings of depression. Relationships, jobs, status, health, money, dignity, and self-esteem are frequently lost as a result of addiction. Depression can also be caused by a relapse to substance use. This is especially true after a significant period of abstinence and recovery.

For many, getting and staying sober helps decrease or eliminate feelings of depression. This is not true for everyone, however. Some still feel depressed even after being sober for weeks or months. Yet others experience depression long after getting sober from substances.

Some people have a type of clinical depression that is more than the blues or feeling down that everyone experiences from time to time. This condition is referred to as *major depression* and requires professional treatment. People with substance use disorders have higher rates of major depression than the general population.

Major depression involves experiencing symptoms nearly every day, for two weeks or longer. Symptoms include: feeling depressed, being unable to experience pleasure, loss of appetite, decrease in sexual desire or energy, difficulty concentrating, significant weight change, problems falling asleep, staying asleep or sleeping too much, feeling agitated or restless, feeling hopeless, helpless, worthless, or guilty, or even feeling like life is not worth living or making an actual suicide attempt. For some, depressive symptoms have been more or less present for months or longer.

Major depression is a recurrent condition for over half of the people who experience an episode of it. About 70 percent of people who have had two separate episodes of major depression and 90 percent of those who have had three separate episodes will have a recurrence.[3] This is called *recurrent major depression*. This type of depression requires ongoing use of medications even when symptoms are no longer present. Medicine reduces the likelihood of a future recurrence.

Some people have a chronic, low grade type of depression called *dysthymia*. This persists for years. It can also co-occur with major depression (called double depression in this case). Others have a *seasonal* pattern and are more prone to depression at certain times of the year such as winter. Some women who have children experience *post-partum depression* after they deliver their baby. Finally, depression is also common with anxiety, eating, and personality disorders.

Even if you don't have depressive illness you can benefit from learning new ways to handle feelings of depression so your recovery goes better.

Recovery Activity

1. Which of the following symptoms of depression have you been experiencing in the past month?

    ❑ Feeling depressed, sad, down in the dumps, blue

    ❑ Trouble experiencing pleasure

    ❑ Poor appetite

- ❏ Poor sleep (can't fall asleep, awake during night, wake up too early and don't feel rested)
- ❏ Feeling irritated or agitated
- ❏ Feeling slowed down, hard to get motivated or moving to do things
- ❏ Difficulty concentrating or remembering things
- ❏ Feeling helpless, hopeless or guilty
- ❏ Loss of, or decrease in sexual desire
- ❏ Thoughts that life isn't worth living or wanting to commit suicide
- ❏ Having a plan to take your own life
- ❏ Actually made a suicide attempt

2. How much of a problem is depression for you?
   ❏ No problem ❏ Small problem ❏ Moderate problem ❏ Serious problem

3. Depression has affected my life in the following ways: _____

   _____

   _____

4. Problems contributing to my depression include: _____

   _____

   _____

5. I tend to have a lot of negative, pessimistic, or depressing thoughts about myself or the future.
   ❏ Yes ❏ No Explain your answer:

   _____

   _____

   _____

6. My use of alcohol or drugs affects my depression in the following ways:

   _____

   _____

   _____

Strategies for Managing Depression

1. **Find out problems causing you to feel depressed and do something about them.** If you feel depressed because you are overweight, then do something about your weight. If you feel depressed because you hate your job, look at other options. If you feel depressed because your relationships are unsatisfying, look for ways to improve these relationships or develop new ones. However, depression is not always related to "problems" or "life events." Sometimes, biological factors may be the primary factor contributing to depression. This is especially true of people who have two or more episodes of clinical depression. This is called *recurrent de-*

pression and having this type of depression increases your chances of having future episodes. Make sure you get a thorough physical examination so that medical causes of depression can be ruled out first.

2. **Evaluate your relationships with other people.** Develop new relationships or improve relationships that are problematic and which contribute to feeling depressed. Look at whether your emotional needs are being satisfied from your current relationships.

3. **Make amends.** Depression can be connected to guilt associated with hurting others because of your alcohol or drug problem. Making amends can help you feel better about yourself. The Twelve-Step program can help guide you through the process of making amends. A counselor or sponsor can help you determine when you are ready to make amends to specific people you feel were hurt by your substance use.

4. **Keep active.** Even if you have to force yourself to do things, keep active in your social relationships, and with your hobbies and interests. When you least want to do things may be when you most need to. Physical activity like walking, running, working out, working around the house or yard, or playing sports may indirectly help improve your depression.

5. **Talk about your feelings and problems with others.** Share your feelings with supportive people such as close friends, family members, a sponsor or counselor. Venting feelings may provide you with some relief and help you gain a different perspective on your depression. Or, you may learn some new ideas on coping with depression from other people. Guard against always talking about your depression with others. People usually are supportive to a degree. If you don't try to help yourself and do some things differently to cope with your depression, others can get tired of hearing you constantly talk about your depressed feelings.

6. **Look for other emotions or feelings that may contribute to, or be associated with, depression.** Other emotions may contribute to feelings of depression. Some people are prone to feeling more depressed when they hold onto feelings of anger. Others may feel depressed if they don't work through guilt and shame. Some people get depressed as a result of constantly feeling anxious or fearful.

7. **Change your depressed thoughts.** Your thoughts can contribute to feelings of depression. Learn to identify and challenge negative, pessimistic or depressed thoughts. Avoid making mountains out of molehills, always looking at the negative side of things, always expecting the worst case scenario or dwelling on your mistakes or shortcomings. Use self-talk strategies to change negative thoughts (i.e., in response to making a mistake, instead of saying "I'm not capable of doing this," say "I made a mistake. It's no big deal, everyone makes mistakes.").

8. **Focus on positive things.** Make sure you acknowledge your positive points or strengths. Don't take yourself for granted, and give yourself credit for your positive qualities. Take an inventory of your achievements or the positive things happening in your life, no matter how small. Learn to look at the "other" side of things when you catch yourself thinking negatively. For example, suppose you lost twenty-five pounds over several months only to gain five back. Rather than put yourself down and feel depressed for gaining the five pounds back, remind yourself you are still twenty pounds down from your previous weight. Remember, sometimes it's not so much what you do but how you think about what you do that determines how you feel.

9. **Keep a journal.** Writing about your feelings can help you release them or better understand them. This can also help you figure out if there are patterns to your feelings and behaviors. For example, suppose you discover that you tend to feel more depressed after visiting your parents. In exploring this further, you discover these feelings relate to constantly being criticized by your father, or because your mother usually is drunk when you visit and this triggers bad feelings and memories. A journal can help you keep track of changes in your depression over time as well as the positive coping strategies that seem to help the most. In addition, write about positive or hopeful things that happen to you each day.

10. **Participate in pleasant activities each day.** Put some time aside each day to do something that is fun, enjoyable, or pleasurable. Even small things like taking fifteen minutes for yourself each day to read a magazine and enjoy a cup of coffee or tea may help you feel better.

11. **Identify and plan future activities that you can look forward to enjoying.** We all need things to look forward to, whether it is buying something nice for ourselves, taking a vacation, or participating in an enjoyable activity. Having things to look forward to breaks up the monotony of doing the same old things over and over. It provides a focus for your energy and can make you feel invested in life. Set some goals in relation to activities, events, or experiences that you can plan and look forward to.

12. **If your depression doesn't get better, seek a mental health evaluation.** If your depression continues and causes personal suffering or interferes with your life, seek an evaluation with a mental health professional. There are many different types of treatment that are effective for clinical depression. These include various types of therapy as well as the use of antidepressant medications. Not all clinical depressions need medications. But if yours does, you should not feel guilty. It is not the same as drinking alcohol or using drugs to get high or loaded. For some people, clinical depression is a chronic disorder requiring ongoing treatment (recurrent depression or dysthymia). If you have had two or more episodes of depression you probably need ongoing treatment, even after your depression improves or lifts completely. People who stop treatment for depression put themselves at risk for relapse in the future.

20. Expressing Positive Emotions

The four previous sections of this workbook reviewed emotions or feelings associated with distress or suffering that can lead to addiction relapse such as anger, anxiety, boredom or depression. Keep in mind it is not the emotion or feeling that determines whether you relapse, but whether you use coping skills to manage emotions.

Sharing and expressing emotions or feelings such as affection, love, joy, and happiness are also important in recovery.[1] Sharing positive feelings can bring you closer to others and improve your relationships. There should be a balance in your life in expressing negative and positive emotions.

For example, we all need love in our lives. Feeling loved and cared about, and loving and caring about others can bring fulfillment to our lives. Having loving relationships with others is one of the most basic of all human needs and enriches our lives.

On the other hand, a lack of loving relationships, an inability to express or show love toward others, or an inability to actually feel love toward others causes you to feel bad, depressed, lonely, or empty. Psychiatric, substance use and co-occurring disorders can harm love relationships. Recovery, on the other hand, provides opportunities to restore loving relationships and develop new ones.

Although you may think about love as a feeling or emotion, it is much more. It is also an attitude and approach to others and to life. Love involves your behaviors or what you say and do. With love, similar to other emotions, actions speak louder than words. How you treat others reveals your emotions more than what you say to them. For instance, you can tell another person how much you care about and love them, but treat them shabbily. Or, you may seldom tell another that you love or care for them, but treat them with much kindness, respect, and love in your actions.

Gratitude is another example of a positive feeling.[2] This refers to feeling thankful or having appreciation to others (or God) for actions of others, your relationship with others or other "gifts" in life (e.g., good health, creative talents, opportunities).

This section of the workbook will help you examine positive emotions. It will review some strategies to express love and other positive emotions in your life.

Recovery Activity

1. How often do you express positive emotions toward others?
   ❑ Regularly ❑ Frequently ❑ Occasionally ❑ Seldom

2. How difficult is it for you to express love or other positive emotions?
   ❑ Very difficult ❑ Difficult ❑ Somewhat ❑ Not at all

3. If you have difficulty expressing positive emotions, describe the reasons.

   _____

   _____

4. What would you like to change about the frequency or way in which you express positive emotions to others?

   _____

   _____

   _____

   _____

Strategies to Express Positive Emotions

1. **Spend time with people important to you.** Time with family and close friends is one of the most precious gifts you can give. Show love for your parents, spouse, children, or close friends by spending time with them. Don't use the excuse of being too busy as a reason not to take time to be with those important to you.

2. **Take an active interest in the lives of loved ones.** Ask your loved ones about their lives and what is important to them. Ask them about their daily activities at home, work, and school; what they think about things going on in the family or in the world; and about their hobbies or interests. Find out what excites them, and about their hopes and dreams.

3. **Do nice things for others.** Help others with a problem or task such as cleaning the house, yard work, homework or something else. Offer to take them out for a meal, to a movie, or other event, or to do something you know interests them. Honor special occasions (birthdays, graduations, mother's day, father's day, etc.) or surprise your loved one with an unexpected gift, card, or personal note.

4. **Attend to the needs of people important to you.** Close, loving relationships require an ability to give and take. "Giving" means being aware of what the other person needs and trying your best to meet those needs. For example, if your partner needs time to talk about her day, give her time and show interest in what she says. If your partner has the need to do things that you do not enjoy, compromise and do some of these things together. If your son or daughter needs attention and reassurance of your love, convey this in your words and actions.

5. **Make positive statements to others.** Say nice things to others. This can be about something they said or did. Or, it can be a reminder that you value, admire, appreciate, or love them. Or, you can let them know you are grateful they are part of your life or that you enjoy being with them.

6. **Do a gratitude inventory.** Make a list of people you feel grateful to have in your life and write about why you are grateful. Include in your inventory a list of "gifts" for which you feel grateful. Gifts can be physical, mental, emotional, creative, spiritual, or relate to any area of your life.

7. **Show love and gratitude through physical gestures or gifts.** Touching, hugging, or kissing are ways to show your positive feelings to people you love such as a family member or intimate partner. Also, giving gifts (even small ones) is an excellent way to convey your affection and love for another person.

8. **Do not let emotional baggage accumulate.** Dealing with upsetting feelings directly, so they do not build up, makes it easier to share love toward others. Therefore, do not let anger or disappointment toward a loved one build up because it can interfere with your desire to share love or other positive feelings. If you are married or live with your intimate partner, never go to bed angry. Work things out first. However, make sure you communicate in respectful ways. Do not attack, use hostility or contempt, or put the other person down when discussing your anger or upset feelings because this will only make things worse. In the event you say some things you think you should have not said during a discussion, apologize and work hard to avoid this in the future.

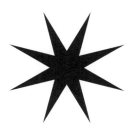

SECTION V

Relationships and Support Systems

21. My Family and Recovery

Families are often affected by psychiatric illness, substance abuse, or co-occurring disorders.[1–3] Mood or atmosphere, communication, how members get along and financial conditions are just a few examples of the areas of family life that are affected. In addition, the physical, emotional, and spiritual health of individual members can also be affected. An important aspect of recovery is to understand how your family was actually affected by your co-occurring disorders and encourage them to get involved in recovery if needed. Some of the common concerns and questions of families include the following:

1. **Understanding illness and treatment:** families want to know what your disorders are and what caused them. They want to know how long you might have to be in treatment, how it can help you and what should be done if treatment doesn't seem to work. They may be concerned with how long you will have to take medicines, what side-effects you may experience and what may happen if you drink alcohol or use drugs when you're on medications for a psychiatric disorder.

2. **Responsibility:** families are often concerned about where their responsibility ends and yours begins in relation to your recovery. Sometimes families worry about doing too much for you and taking over too many of your responsibilities.

3. **Family role in treatment:** families wonder to what degree they should get involved in your treatment. Some worry about getting blamed for your problems. Members also wonder whether they need help themselves to cope with their reactions and feelings.

4. **Other family members getting sick:** with psychiatric illness in particular, families are often concerned that if one member has an illness another person may get sick as well. Many disorders run in families making members feel vulnerable.

5. **Threat of loss:** family members worry that they may lose the member with co-occurring disorders, particularly when this person is a parent. They sometimes feel deprived of their time, attention and love. This is especially true in cases when the disorder is so severe that you aren't emotionally available to your family or unable to take care of your family.

6. **Threat to security:** family members worry about their physical, emotional and psychological security especially when a parent is the one with co-occurring disorders. If your behaviors include violence or poor judgment when you do things to threaten the security of your family, they are likely to feel even more insecure.

7. **Long-term outcome:** another typical concern of families relates to the worry they have about the long-term outcome of treatment. They wonder how your disorders and participation in recovery may affect you in the long-term. This is particularly true if you have been in the hospital many times or have had serious life problems as a result of your disorders.

8. **Financial burden:** the cost of treatment, cost associated with the legal system, and loss of income related to being able to keep a job or find a job often can create a financial burden on the family. If, as a parent, your alcohol or drug use or your psychiatric symptoms led to you being unable to work and provide for your family, financial problems probably occurred.

9. **Emotional burden:** families often feel emotionally drained, tired, or burned out from dealing with co-occurring disorders and related behaviors. In some cases they may have symptoms of psychiatric illness themselves, such as a serious mood disorder or serious anxiety disorder. Or, family members may have their own alcohol or drug problems.

10. **Effectiveness of treatment:** families worry whether treatment will help you since relapse rates are high with chronic psychiatric illness and addiction. If you have been in multiple treatments and have been on a number of different medications over the years and you still show symptoms, your family is more likely to worry about you.

11. **Lack of motivation to get well:** since many people with co-occurring disorders don't admit their problems or seek help, families worry about how to encourage their ill member to get help. Once the dual diagnosis member is in treatment, families may worry about how to deal with any lack of motivation their member may have to work their recovery program and make positive changes.

12. **Suicide risk:** suicide attempts and threats are stressful to families. Families worry about whether or not they can detect suicidal thinking and do anything about it.

13. **Relapse:** another concern is whether or not you'll get sick again with the symptoms of your psychiatric illness. If you've had multiple episodes of illness over time or a chronic course of illness, your family may worry about your symptoms coming back or getting worse. Since alcohol and drugs cause so many problems within the family, members worry whether or not you'll use again. This is especially true if you've been in recovery before and have relapsed several times.

14. **Hospitalization:** families worry about whether or not hospitalization is needed in certain cases where your symptoms return or your alcohol or drug use gets out of control. Families are concerned about how to get you into the hospital when you resist and refuse to go along with their recommendations to get help in the hospital. If your behavior is a serious threat to yourself or others and they have to hospitalize you involuntarily, families may feel guilty for doing this.

Try to put yourself in your family's shoes so you can understand what coping with your alcohol and drug problem and your psychiatric disorder has been like from their point of view. This may lead you to a greater understanding of their experiences.

Recovery Activity

1. Describe below how you think your family has been affected by your disorders.

    _____

    _____

    _____

2. Describe how your spouse or partner has been affected by your disorders.

    _____

    _____

    _____

3. Describe how your children have been affected by your disorders.

    _____

    _____

    _____

4. Describe how other family members have been affected by your disorders.

    _____

    _____

    _____

5. Have any of your family members expressed concerns about your alcohol or other drug use or your psychiatric condition? If yes, what did they tell you?

    _____

    _____

    _____

At some point in recovery, consider "making amends" to your family for the difficulties caused by your disorders. Who, when and how to do this are issues to discuss with your therapist or sponsor. While you don't want to rush into this too quickly, you must also guard against putting it off.

You can begin this process by getting your family involved in recovery if possible, and by making sure you spend time with them. It is helpful to sit down and talk face-to-face with family members and hear from them what it was like, and how they felt about both your addiction and your psychiatric disorder. However, since not all family members are able, willing, or even should be involved in recovery, this is an issue you should discuss first with your therapist or sponsor. A therapist can help you determine what to do about this issue. There are instances when the harm has been so great, that directly making amends to a family member is not advised. Participating in family therapy is often helpful in addressing some of these important issues in recovery.

Example #1: Nicole's Effect on Her Family and Her Plan

"My depression, hurting myself and threatening suicide too many times to count, and abuse of alcohol and drugs has really hurt my parents a lot. I've done about everything to my parents that you could imagine one could do including lying to them, threatening to hurt myself, getting high and saying nasty things to their face, and basically just being rotten to them. Since I've been in and out of psych hospitals and rehab programs, outpatient counseling and AA and NA too many times to count, I know that my words to them will be shallow if they are not backed up with a plan. Frankly, I know they're probably tired of me making verbal amends to them only to go out and do the same things over and over. I guess you could say it's been an emotional and a financial strain on my parents. And my sister, she basically washed her hands of me. I've said a lot of bad things to her as well as stormed over to her apartment on many occasions when I've either been high or upset with someone. It's not going to be easy, but I know what I have to do to get closer to my family. The first and most important thing is that I have to stay in treatment. I have to stay on my medication, go to therapy and not miss appointments, and go to my NA meetings. There are no ifs, ands, or buts about any of this. I also have talked to my doctor and my outpatient therapist and we have agreed that I'm going to bring my parents to sessions every month. This way, we can talk about my progress as well as any problems I'm having. We can also talk about what's realistic for them in terms of how they can help me as well as what I need to do myself. My parents have always stood beside me and probably have done too much for me in the past. In some ways I guess you could say that they have to get a little tougher on me. The bottom line is that if we work together, there is a greater chance that I can do better in my recovery and improve things with my family."

Your Children

Sometimes, children in families where a parent has a psychiatric disorder, alcohol or drug abuse problem or both, develop serious problems themselves. These may be emotional, behavioral, school, or alcohol and drug problems. If any of your children show the symptoms or problems below, arrange to have them evaluated by a mental health professional to determine if treatment is needed.

- Severe anxiety, depression or mood swings
- Hears voices or has very bizarre thoughts or ideas (i.e., that people are trying to put thoughts in or take them out of their head)
- Becomes violent with other people
- Expresses thoughts of suicide
- Has trouble sitting still, concentrating or completing school work leading to poor grades
- Skips school a lot, has trouble getting along with other kids at home or school
- Has trouble with rules or breaks the law

If any of your children are using alcohol or drugs, arrange to have them evaluated by a drug or alcohol treatment professional.

Children benefit from participating in support groups such as Alateen or treatment sessions with a therapist. If you have any concerns about how your children may have been affected by your co-occurring disorders, ask your social worker or other members of your treatment team what services may be available for them. When children learn about co-occurring disorders, it helps them better understand what their parent has gone through.

In your opinion, do any of your children need an evaluation for a possible mental health problem or alcohol/drug use problem?　　❑　Yes　❑　No

If yes, what steps can you take to get your child an assessment or treatment?

_____

_____

Example #2: Daryl's Effects on His Son and His Plan

"I know my addiction and my crazy-ass behavior really messed up my family. My nine-year-old son, Daryl, is having a lot of trouble. He gets in fights all the time at school, sasses the teacher, and doesn't do what he is told. He has trouble getting along with his brothers and sisters, too. My son, Daryl even sasses me and doesn't listen to me sometimes. Things seem to be getting worse instead of better. Even though I'm doing better and I'm in recovery now, my son Daryl is still having trouble. So me and my wife decided that we need to get him seen to figure out if he needs treatment, too. I talked this over with my outpatient therapist and we made an arrangement for him to get an evaluation and for the family to be seen as well. This way we can figure out if any kind of treatment will be needed for Daryl. Ain't no doubt in my mind that the boy needs help. This is the time to do it now."

22. Saying No to Getting High

One of the most common factors contributing to relapse to alcohol or drug use is pressure from other people to use substances.[1, 2] Pressures may be direct, with other people offering you *substances* or inviting you to use or party with them. Pressures may also be indirect and occur when you are in situations where other people are using but aren't asking you directly to use *substances* with them. Parties, work functions, graduations, weddings and other social events are just some activities where people may be drinking alcohol and not offering any to you directly. By thinking ahead and identifying the social pressures you are likely to experience in figuring out some way to refuse offers to get high, you put yourself in a better position to keep your sobriety.

When you're in a situation where you feel direct or indirect pressure to use chemicals, sometimes it taps a part of you that still wants to get high. As a result, you may feel anxious, worried or even excited. It is not unusual to have mixed feelings—where part of you wants to give in to the pressure to use and part of you doesn't. Remember, even though you may want to use doesn't mean you have to use. Therefore, you have to be prepared with some ways to say no to drugs or alcohol and get out of situations where you experience very strong pressure to get high.

You also need to be able to identify people that you have a relationship with who pose a threat to your ongoing sobriety. These are people who want to get high with you, or who want to use while they're around you. For example, if you are trying to stay clean from cocaine or alcohol and your partner or spouse gets high when around you, this creates pressure than may increase your risk for relapse. It can be hard to stay straight when others around you are getting high in front of you. If your close relationships involve people who get high and have a drug or alcohol problem, you're going to have to figure out ways of coping with this to protect your own recovery. Talk this over with your therapist, doctor and sponsor in self-help programs. While these social pressures can create stress for you, if you use positive coping skills you can avoid relapse.

Recovery Activity

1. List people who are likely to directly invite you to use alcohol or drugs or likely to use while they are around you and make you feel pressure to get high.

    _____

    _____

    _____

2. Imagine you're being offered alcohol or drugs right now.
    What *feelings* does this trigger?

    _____

    _____

    What *thoughts* does this trigger?

    _____

    _____

3. Imagine you're offered your drug of choice by one of the people listed above. State how you could refuse this offer and protect your sobriety.

_____

_____

4. If you imagine yourself giving in to the social pressure to use alcohol or other drugs, how is this likely to affect you?

5. Imagine yourself successfully refusing the offer to get high and state how this will affect you as well. *Example: "I'll feel good about myself for making the right decision to stay sober."*

_____

_____

Strategies to Cope with Pressures to Get High

1. **Say no:** state straight out that you don't want to use alcohol or drugs.

2. **Focus on recovery:** tell the person offering you that you are in recovery and don't want to use substances.

3. **Medications:** tell the person you are on medication and can't drink alcohol or use other drugs while taking this.

4. **Leave the situation:** get out of the situation as quickly as you can if you feel increased pressure to use.

5. **Use a support person:** if there is an upcoming event you cannot miss, like a wedding of a family member, take a support person with you.

Coping with Pressures to Stop Taking Your Medicine

Some people in recovery will be pressured by others in recovery to stop taking medications. You may be made to feel guilty or led to believe that taking medication for a psychiatric disorder means that you're not sober or clean as part of your recovery. Don't believe this for a minute because taking medication for a psychiatric illness doesn't mean that you're not in recovery. In fact, not taking the medication is more likely to increase your risk of relapse. Remember, other people can't play doctor and if you're on medication for a psychiatric illness then you need to continue to take it. If any person tries to convince you to get off your medication, don't give in to this pressure.

Many have found it helpful to think about this ahead of time and devise some ways they would cope with pressures to get off medication. In the spaces below write down two or more examples of how you could respond if another person tells you to quit taking your medication.

_____

_____

_____

_____

23. Developing and Using a Support System

No one can recover alone. It is important to develop and use a support system as part of your recovery.[1,2] A support system consists of people in your life that can help you and support your recovery. These are people you can lean on during rough times or who are important in your life.

Your support system usually involves professionals who provide your treatment. That includes AA, NA, Dual Recovery Anonymous (DRA), or Double Trouble in Recovery (DTR) support group sponsors or members, close friends and family members. These should be people with whom you have regular contact and with whom you can share your thoughts, feelings and struggles. People in your network ideally are those who also are willing to be honest and tell you if you are slacking off your recovery program or acting in ways that increase the chances of a relapse. People in your recovery network should be ones who will help if you relapse to your psychiatric illness or your addiction.

You can use this network in many ways: for emotional support; to discuss a problem; to discuss thoughts about dropping out of treatment; to talk through strong desires to use alcohol or drugs; or, to share some time together in a social or recreational activity. Regular discussions with members of your network, such as a sponsor or counselor, can help you identify problems early and figure out plans to deal with these before a relapse occurs.

Sometimes, other people will notice relapse warning signs before you do. You may find it helpful to ask members of your support network to point out any warning signs they notice. Keep in mind, however, that it is your responsibility to take action to cope with your warning signs if someone points them out.

Individuals who have a solid support system are more likely than others to maintain their recovery. They are more likely to feel secure because of having a network of people they can rely on for support efforts at recovery and help with problems.

Your Support Network

1. List the names, phone numbers and/or e-mail addresses of people whom you can rely on for support and help in recovering from co-occurring disorders.

    _____

    _____

    _____

    _____

    _____

    _____

2.   Do you have a sponsor in AA, NA or DRA? __Yes __ No. List ways a sponsor can help you.

_____

_____

_____

3.   List ways that members of your support network can help you.

_____

_____

_____

_____

_____

Strategies to Use Your Support Network

1.   **Make a list of people or organizations to include in your support network.** Keep this list handy and make a copy to keep on you at all times so you always have it. Write this list on a card or piece of paper you can put in your wallet or purse. Or, put it in your cell phone so you have easy access to it.

2.   **Accept recovery as a "we" program.** You need to rely on others for help and support. Identify people you can depend on who will support your recovery. Don't rely only on yourself.

3.   **Reach out to others for help and support.** Don't wait for others to read your mind. Tell yourself it is OK to ask others for help or support. Overcome your reluctance to ask others for help and support. When you least want to reach out for help and support may be the time in which you need to reach out.

4.   **Get a sponsor in your Twelve-Step program.** Talk with this person every day. Let them teach you the ropes about recovery. Listen to what they have to say. "Work" the Twelve Steps with your sponsor as a way of changing your life and enhancing your recovery.

5.   **Talk to friends in recovery every day.** Stay connected to peers in recovery by talking on the phone, via text messaging or e-mail, or face-to-face.

24. AA/NA/DRA, Mental Health Support Groups, and Recovery Clubs

Participation in mutual support recovery programs offers many benefits. [1,2] Your recovery will go better if you take advantage of support programs available in your community. Your treatment team can help you figure out which mutual support programs or recovery clubs to use, how to get a sponsor in a Twelve-Step program, and what other resources to use.

AA/NA/DRA/DTR Meetings

AA, NA, Dual Recovery Anonymous (DRA), and Double Trouble in Recovery (DTR) offer ongoing support for recovery from addiction or co-occurring disorders. There are different kinds of meetings. A *lead meeting* involves a person sharing his/her story of addiction and recovery. A *discussion meeting* allows all present to share their ideas and experiences related to the topic(s) under discussion. Some meetings are "closed" and available only to those with alcohol or drug problems. Others are "open" and can be attended by anyone. There are many meetings for "select" groups of people such as business people, health care professionals, gay men or lesbian women, young people, newcomers to AA/NA, and other groups. By checking around and attending different meetings, you should be able to find some that you feel can help you. If you are new to the program, attend at least 12 meetings before you judge their usefulness.

Some meetings are for people with co-occurring disorders. These "dual recovery" meetings provide a chance to talk about both your psychiatric illness and your alcohol/drug abuse. Recovery meetings that focus on co-occurring disorders go by a lot of different names. Some examples include: Double Trouble in Recovery, MISA, CAMI, SAMI, and dual recovery. While many people with co-occurring disorders feel that traditional AA/NA meetings benefit them, others prefer going to these special meetings, or to DRA or DTR meetings as well.

The Twelve Steps of AA/NA/DRA

The "Twelve-Step program" of AA/NA/DRA offers an excellent mechanism to make positive changes and stay sober. The steps focus on more than alcohol or drug use. They focus on emotional, personal and spiritual change and growth.

Other Support Groups for Addiction

Some communities have other types of support groups to help in recovery from alcohol or drug problems. Some local support programs you may wish to learn more about to determine if they can help you include Women for Sobriety (WFS), Rational Recovery (RR), and SMART Recovery. Ask your treatment team for more information.

Mental Health Support Programs

Programs like Emotions Anonymous, Emotional Health Anonymous, and Recovery International are also available for people with mental health problems. Some areas have groups for those with specific psychiatric disorders such as depression, bipolar disorder, schizophrenia, or other disorders. These provide a chance to learn about mental health problems and recovery from them. Similar to AA/NA/DRA/DTR meetings, people share hope, strength, and experience and help each other out.

Family Support Programs

These include Al-Anon or Nar-Anon which relate specifically to coping with alcohol and drug abuse in the family and groups related to psychiatric illness and the family such as those sponsored by the National Alliance for the Mentally Ill (NAMI). I recommend that your family attends family programs if possible. They can learn about illness, recovery and how to cope with their own feelings. Family groups provide families with a chance to get support from others and discuss their own concerns.

Sponsorship

A "sponsor" is a person in a Twelve-Step program who has established a solid period of recovery (usually a couple of years or longer). A sponsor helps newcomers learn to use the "tools" of recovery. A sponsor can help in many ways: attending meetings with you, being available for daily discussions on the phone, helping you work the Twelve Steps, being there for you during difficult times and celebrating your successes in recovery.

You can get a sponsor in several ways: ask a member at a meeting who you know has some good recovery time to sponsor you; ask the chairperson at a meeting to help you find a sponsor; call AA/NA/DRA/DTR and ask them if they can help you get a sponsor; or ask a staff member to help you find a sponsor.

Recovery Literature

There is a lot of information available to help you better understand addiction, mental health, co-occurring disorders and recovery. This includes pamphlets, workbooks, books, and electronic media. Ask your therapist, another member of your treatment team, or your sponsor for specific recommendations. Some of the written materials were developed by people like yourself who are recovering from an addiction, mental health, or co-occurring disorders. Other materials were developed by professionals on the following topics: AA, NA, sponsorship, the Twelve Steps, depression, anxiety, anger, specific psychiatric disorders, relapse, alcohol and other drugs, family recovery, and other topics.

Recovery Clubs

Recovery is a process that takes time. The weeks and months after rehab or inpatient treatment is a critical time period in recovery. Fill your time with positive, constructive activities to replace time previously spent using substances. Avoid negative people, places and things that trigger a desire to get high and hinder your recovery program.

The idea of recovery clubs came about as a way of helping fill time in a constructive way. All have the same purpose for those recovering from addiction—to provide a safe environment where you can meet and talk with other recovering people, attend meetings, and share ideas about the process of recovery. Most recovery clubs have recreational activities such as pool tables, ping pong tables and places one can play cards. While doing these activities, you are in a constructive atmosphere that promotes openness and honesty, which is important throughout recovery.

The hours of operation vary from club to club but usually the hours are from early morning until late at night if not beyond midnight on the weekends. Many of the clubs sponsor dances, picnics, and periodic large social events that are attended by many people from support groups such as NA, Al-Anon, Adult Children Anonymous (ACA), CA, and Gamblers Anonymous (GA).

Food is also available at a nominal cost for the people attending recovery clubs. The quality of food is not gourmet by any standard, but it is very moderately priced and provides a place where you can go and have breakfast, lunch, or dinner in a safe environment where there are no chemicals.

Recovery Activity

1. Check the following types of programs you participate in.
    ___AA/NA meetings   ___DRA or dual recovery   ___Mental health related

2. List any reservations you have about participating in mutual support programs.

    _____

    _____

    _____

    _____

3. List ways that you think these support programs can help you.

    _____

    _____

    _____

4. List benefits of working the Twelve-Step program of AA/NA.

    _____

    _____

    _____

5. List ways a sponsor can help you.

    _____

    _____

    _____

6. List benefits of reading recovery literature on a regular basis.

    _____

    _____

    _____

7. List benefits of spending time in a recovery club.

    _____

    _____

    _____

8. If you feel like cutting down or stopping your involvement in support programs, what should you do BEFORE making a final decision?

_____

_____

_____

Step 1 Worksheet

1. In your own words, state what you think Step 1 means:

   _____

   _____

   _____

   _____

   _____

2. Give some examples of your own powerlessness over alcohol or drugs:

   (1) _____

   (2) _____

   (3) _____

   (4) _____

   (5) _____

   (6) _____

3. Give some examples of how your alcohol and drug use led to unmanageability in your life:

   (1) _____

   (2) _____

   (3) _____

   (4) _____

   (5) _____

   (6) _____

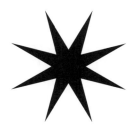

SECTION VI

Changing
the Self

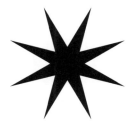

25. Changing Self-Defeating and Self-Destructive Behaviors

Self-defeating behaviors are actions that hurt your physical, emotional, social or spiritual health, relationships and ability to function as a responsible adult. Patterns of self-defeating behavior can show in the way you relate to other people, cope with problems or stress, or deal with taking care of your basic needs and obligations. Examples of self-defeating patterns of relationship behaviors include jumping from one relationship to the next, getting easily bored and leaving your partner, getting involved in relationships with people who do not take care of your needs and are abusive to you, or getting into a relationship when you have little in common with the other person and are likely to become dissatisfied with this relationship. Some self-defeating patterns are obvious. Others are less obvious and you have to look closely at your life to see if they are present. *Self-destructive behaviors* are those that threaten serious harm to you. These behaviors also pose a risk to any area of your health or well-being. These include compulsive behaviors such as alcohol or drug dependence, compulsive gambling, overeating or sex. Other self-destructive behaviors include attempts to hurt yourself or take your own life through a suicidal gesture or putting yourself in danger by driving a car recklessly, engaging in risky sexual behaviors, acting aggressively or violently toward others.

Recovery Activity

1. Following are examples of self-destructive and self-defeating behaviors. Check the ones that concern you at this time in your recovery.
   - ❑ Making suicidal threats or gestures.
   - ❑ Being too controlling with others.
   - ❑ Jumping from one relationship to the next.
   - ❑ Getting easily bored with my partner.
   - ❑ Moving in with a partner who I have known for only a short period of time.
   - ❑ Purposely saying things that hurt other people.
   - ❑ Holding feelings inside and not communicating directly to others.
   - ❑ Letting people take advantage of me and holding onto my resentments.
   - ❑ Picking up strangers or people I don't know and having sex with them.
   - ❑ Not using protection for sex; sex with strangers or multiple partners.
   - ❑ Getting involved too quickly in a romantic relationship.
   - ❑ Cheating on my spouse or intimate partner.
   - ❑ Not spending time with my children or family members.
   - ❑ Getting involved in a relationship that is physically or emotionally abusive.
   - ❑ Using intimidation and anger to keep people away from me or on guard.
   - ❑ Conning others and scamming to get money or taking advantage of them.
   - ❑ Hanging out with others who are getting high on alcohol or drugs.
   - ❑ Getting into fights or hurting other people through violence.
   - ❑ Not being responsible at work or school (missing, late, not doing work).

- ❏ Not sticking with a job, quitting a job impulsively or too many different jobs.
- ❏ Managing my money poorly and getting deep into debt.
- ❏ Spending money I need for basic necessities on things I don't need.
- ❏ Starting projects or jobs and not finishing them.
- ❏ Not setting any goals or having any sense of direction in my life.
- ❏ Making mistakes but blaming bad fortune or others for these.
- ❏ Not having structure, routine or direction in my life.
- ❏ Not following through with my medical treatment or medical advice.
- ❏ Not following through with treatment for either of my co-occurring disorders.
- ❏ Continuing to get high on alcohol or other drugs.
- ❏ Keeping alcohol or drugs in my home in order to test myself.
- ❏ Compulsive behaviors: gambling, sex, overeating, Internet use, spending.
- ❏ Eating and then making myself vomit.
- ❏ Cutting, burning, or damaging my body.
- ❏ Spending too much time watching TV, playing videos or on the computer.
- ❏ Spending too much idle time and being unproductive.
- ❏ Getting involved in too many projects or activities.
- ❏ Spending too much time at work or working at home.
- ❏ Getting involved in illegal activities or criminal behaviors.
- ❏ Other behaviors that cause me problems (write in below).

_____

_____

_____

2. Choose one behavior from this list that you would like to change and write it below. Then, write down several steps you can take to change this behavior.

_____

_____

_____

_____

_____

The first step in changing behaviors is identifying those that are a problem. The above examples should help you begin to identify which behaviors you may need to change. The next step is figuring out a specific plan of action to help you change one or more of your patterns of behavior. Use the following examples to guide you in beginning to look at how you can change one behavior.

Example #1: Shauntey's Self-Defeating Relationship Pattern

"I have a long pattern of getting hooked up with men who take advantage of me. They use me for sex and get money and drugs from me. A couple guys have even beat me up, but I stuck with them because I didn't want to be alone and thought I could change them. I'm working on changing this relationship pattern. The first thing I have to do is go slow in developing any new relationships with men. I can no longer let myself get sexually and emotionally involved with men that I hardly know because I always end up getting used and hurt. Also, there's no way I can get involved with a man who gets high because I'm too vulnerable and likely to let him drag me down. I'll work on developing friendships first. Then, if any other type of relationship follows, I'll be in better shape emotionally to handle it."

Example #2: Rob's Self-Destructive Pattern of Aggressiveness

"For years I've been getting into fights. I can't tell you how many people I messed up or how many times my ass has been whipped. My pattern has been to retaliate and "get even" with anyone who does me wrong. I never even cared if I got hurt. Shit, I not only been beat up real bad, but I even got stabbed twice. It didn't use to matter to me 'cause I ain't never been scared of no one. But, I'm getting too old for this shit. I'm tired of the streets and fighting.

First thing I need to do is to stay off all drugs and alcohol. I gotta change my nasty attitude and stop gettin' in peoples' faces to create trouble. I been in jail a couple times and the forensic unit of a mental hospital once and I had enough. I got two kids who are doing real good and I want to see them get to college 'cause I ain't never finished high school. If I still live with the street mentality I just ain't gonna make it. It's just a matter of time. A real key is going to therapy and NA meetings and sticking with them 'cause in the past, I always stop when I hear the truth from a therapist or sponsor about my attitude and nastiness."

Example #3: Jenny's Poor Money Management

"I make good money, but I got myself deep in debt because of my cocaine use and poor money management. Now that I am off drugs, I'm making some changes and doing good. But, it's hard to resist my desire to buy whatever I want. I consolidated my credit cards to get a lower payment and interest rate. I'm following a budget where I pay bills, put money in an IRA retirement fund and save money before doing anything else. I now budget money for clothes whereas before, I bought whatever I wanted by using credit cards, which led to large credit card balances. Eating out is something I always did, now I do this infrequently, but only if I have money for it. It helps to write down everything I buy so I can track my spending habits. I review my budget at the beginning and end of the month with my boyfriend who is helping me stay focused."

26. Changing Personality Problems

Changing personality problems, which show in your thinking and behavior, is an excellent means of self-improvement.[1] Twelve-Step programs suggest changing "defects of character" as part of your recovery. Many people with psychiatric disorders and addiction have a personality disorder, which refers to having a group of personality traits or behaviors that cause difficulty or considerable distress in life. Even if you don't have a personality disorder, you too can benefit from changing behaviors.

Personality traits refer to the way you view and relate to the world. They show in your attitudes and behaviors, and play a major role in your ability to function in life and get along with others. Since traits are "ingrained," they can be hard to change and it takes time and effort to do so.

Following is a list of traits associated with personality. Some can be seen in terms of "opposites." For each trait, there often is another one that is somewhat of an opposite one. For example, the opposite of "self-centered" is being "other-centered," the opposite of "patient" is "impatient," and the opposite of "perfectionistic" is being "chaotic or scattered." It isn't whether or not you have a particular trait, but the degree to which you have the trait and how it affects your sense of self and your relationships that determine whether or not it is a problem for you.

Recovery Activity

1. Check the following traits or behaviors that describe you.
   - ❑ **Passive:** letting things happen to me without speaking my mind, letting others take advantage of me and holding my thoughts and feelings inside.
   - ❑ **Aggressive:** letting my thoughts and feelings out without regard for others, being pushy with others, or being verbally or physically intrusive.
   - ❑ **Shy and inhibited:** it's hard to talk or share things with others or let others get close. I'm too quiet and wait for others to engage me in conversations.
   - ❑ **Uninhibited:** saying or doing whatever I want without thinking about the impact on others.
   - ❑ **Self-centered:** seeing things mainly from my point of view and not focusing on other people's ideas, feelings, or needs.
   - ❑ **Other-centered:** focusing too much time and energy on taking care of others and meeting their needs, often at the expense of ignoring my own needs.
   - ❑ **Impulsive:** acting before I think about the consequences of my behavior, doing what I want when I want to and doing whatever suits me at the moment.
   - ❑ **Controlling:** wanting to be in control of situations and people and do things my way, and having trouble letting others make decisions or give input.
   - ❑ **Perfectionistic:** wanting things to be "just right," having high expectations, or difficulty allowing myself to make mistakes or fail at something.
   - ❑ **Antisocial:** conning, lying, cheating, taking advantage of, or manipulating others to get what I want, breaking the rules and laws, or not caring about how I affect others.
   - ❑ **Prosocial:** caring about or doing things for others, making a difference in the world and caring about society.

- ❑ **Conscientious:** being concerned about what I do and my impact on other people, wanting to do the right thing or do a good job at whatever I am involved in.
- ❑ **Dependent:** difficulty making decisions on my own and depending too much on others, or having trouble doing things without needing others to guide me.
- ❑ **Independent:** able to make decisions on my own, solve problems, and get my needs satisfied without leaning too much on others.
- ❑ **Cold or aloof:** being detached emotionally from other people, having trouble getting close or sharing positive feelings, or having problems caring for others.
- ❑ **Kind or caring:** giving of myself to others, really caring about what other people do or feel, sharing my time, energy, or resources with others.
- ❑ **Impatient:** having difficulty waiting, wanting things to be done right away, having trouble delaying my needs or gratification, or becoming annoyed with others who move too slowly or who don't do things the way I think they should.
- ❑ **Patient:** able to wait or delay getting my needs satisfied.
- ❑ **Irresponsible:** not taking care of my responsibilities or obligations, not being dependable with others, or doing whatever I want to do.
- ❑ **Overly responsible:** spending too much time and energy making sure things get done and other people get taken care of, worrying too much about things being right, or taking on too many responsibilities.
- ❑ **Suspicious or jealous:** being guarded around others, not trusting their motives, or excessive jealousy.
- ❑ **Insensitive:** not being able to care about or be concerned about the needs and feelings of others, or not caring how I affect them with what I say or do.
- ❑ **Sensitive:** caring about the needs and feelings of others, or trying to understand things from their point of view.
- ❑ **Persistent:** able to stick with things even when the going gets rough. I don't give up easily and keep at things even if it takes hard work or lots of time.
- ❑ **Other (write in):** _____

This is just a partial list of some personality traits and examples of the behavior patterns in which these traits show. There are many other traits as well.

2. Write one item from this list that you would like to change (decrease or control, or increase).

_____

_____

3. List a few steps you can take to begin working on changing this.

_____

_____

_____

_____

Strategies for Changing Behaviors Associated with Personality

1. **Evaluate your traits and behaviors.** You reviewed a list of behaviors associated with personality. Work on changing one thing at a time. Start with something that you want to change and think is possible to change.

2. **Take responsibility for your problems**. Do not blame others or society for your problems, bad luck or circumstances. Own your problems and the need to change.

3. **Change how you think.** Practice new thinking so that you do not act on self-centered, aggressive, hostile or unrealistic thoughts. Learn to challenge your thinking (see next section of workbook for guidance on this area).

4. **Improve your self-control.** Work on controlling your emotions as well as your thinking. Think through problems and options, delay your gratification and anticipate consequences of behaviors before you act.

5. **Work the Twelve Steps and/or use counseling.** A counselor or sponsor can help you take a personal inventory, review your "character defects," and help you target specific behaviors to change. Trust them by opening up and sharing your thoughts, feelings and problems. Do not keep secrets from them.

Example #1: Maria's Need to Control Others

"I'm definitely too controlling and always want things to be my way. I badger my husband all the time to do things that I think he should do. I even try to tell him how to dress. This is going to be real hard to change. But, I can start by cutting down on all the lists I give my husband of things to do around the house. It's like I'm always keeping him busy doing things at home. I can also let him and the children choose recreational activities that they like instead of me being the one who always makes the decision. I can also change this by not making critical remarks about what my husband is wearing when we go out because all this is another way to control him and get him to wear what I think he should wear."

Example #2: Jackson's Tendency to be too Nice and Tolerant of Others

"I'm too nice and tolerant of other people and end up getting taken advantage of as a result. I have to learn how to say no sometimes when other people ask me to do things that I don't want to do. I also have to express my opinion and feelings when people do things that irk me. Like with my brother—he's always late when we decide to go somewhere together and he often borrows money, seldom paying it back on time like he promises. I'm too nice with my kids, too, and let them take advantage of me by getting extra money from me or getting out of doing chores they are supposed to do. I'm going to have to put my foot down because I let resentments build up inside when I let my family or friends take advantage of me. It's not that I want to become hardnosed all the time, it's just that I have to quit being so damn nice all the time."

27. Changing My Thinking

The way you think affects your mood.[1-3] The "internal messages" you give yourself can contribute to feeling anxious, bored, depressed or miserable. Or, these messages can lead to feeling happy, confident and satisfied.

How you think also affects how you act. You can talk yourself into acting in certain ways. For example, you can talk yourself into working hard at your job and succeed as a result of using your self-talk to motivate yourself. Or, you can give yourself messages that you are incompetent and talk yourself into messing up on the job.

Negative or inaccurate thinking can contribute to relapse to alcohol or other drug use. And, it can be a factor in relapse to psychiatric illness.

On the other hand, positive or realistic thinking helps you feel better and improve your relationships and life. Thinking more positively can help you solve problems, feel more confident about your abilities and feel more hopeful about your life. Learning to identify, challenge and reduce negative or inaccurate thinking can lead to positive changes in your moods or behaviors.

Recovery Activity

1. Following are examples of problem thinking associated with co-occurring disorders. Check the statements that represent ways you think about yourself and your life.

    ❏ I make things out to be worse than they really are or make "mountains out of mole-hills."

    ❏ I expect the worst possible thing to happen to me.

    ❏ I often expect to fail at the things I do.

    ❏ I have too many negative thoughts about myself or my life.

    ❏ I focus on the negative side of a situation.

    ❏ I have trouble seeing the positive side of life.

    ❏ I don't think I have many positive qualities or much to offer others.

    ❏ If people knew the real me, they wouldn't like me.

    ❏ I think I'm not capable of getting better.

    ❏ I think I'm not capable of making positive changes in my life.

    ❏ I think I'm not capable of staying off alcohol or other drugs.

    ❏ I keep bothersome thoughts to myself and don't share these with others.

    ❏ I think I need treatment for only a short period of time.

    ❏ I dwell too much on my shortcomings or problems.

    ❏ I worry too much about the future.

    ❏ I think that life isn't worth living (if you feel suicidal, get help right away).

    ❏ I think I can control my alcohol or drug use.

    ❏ I worry I'll hurt someone if I don't control my angry or violent thoughts.

2. Choose two statements from this list and write them below. For each one, list two new, positive or more realistic thoughts.

Thought #1 _____

_____

_____

Two New, Positive Thoughts: _____
(1) _____

_____

(2) _____

_____

Thought #2 _____

_____

_____

Two New, Positive Thoughts: _____
(1) _____

_____

(2) _____

_____

Strategies to Counter Negative Thoughts

Changing thinking takes time and practice like other recovery tasks. Following are some suggested strategies that may help decrease your negative thinking and increase your positive thinking.

1. **Be aware of your negative thought patterns.** Catch yourself when you are thinking negatively. This puts you in a position to challenge and change them.

2. **Challenge negative thinking by checking the evidence.** When you make a statement such as "I'm not capable of change," make sure you check to see what evidence you have that this is true. Often you will find that it is not true in all situations. Even if it is difficult to change, this doesn't mean you can't change. Or, suppose you say to yourself "I'm a failure." If you check all of the evidence, what you would find is that like everyone else you have made mistakes and had failures, but you have also succeeded at things. Negative thinking tends to distort the "big picture" so checking out the facts and the evidence helps you make a "reality check."

3. **Practice positive thinking every day.** Focus on increasing positive thoughts each day by giving yourself messages such as "I'm going to have a good day," or "I'm going to enjoy myself," "I can cope with my problems," or "I have problems, but I have a lot of things going well for me, too." Even if you have to "force" yourself to say nice things or positive things each day, do so.

4. **Focus less on the negative and more on the positive side of a situation.** Instead of seeing the glass as "half empty" and focusing on the negative side of things, look at the other side. Remind yourself of the positive. For example, suppose your AA/NA sponsor or a family member gave you critical feedback about how you were setting yourself up to relapse. Instead of having negative thoughts you might say "It's hard to hear the truth, but they were right in what they said to me. Just because they criticized me doesn't mean I'm not capable of doing OK or that I'm a bad person. It also doesn't mean they are jerks because they told me something that was hard to hear."

5. **Allow room for mistakes.** Don't expect perfection or not to make mistakes. Learn from your mistakes instead of using them to make you feel guilty or incompetent. It is common to make mistakes when trying new behaviors or skills. Learning to think more positively and less negatively is no exception, so give yourself room for error.

6. **Review your progress and accomplishments.** When having a rough time, this can help you see the "bigger picture." Even if things don't always go well, that doesn't mean you don't deserve to compliment yourself for your efforts. Look for even small steps toward change and don't expect major changes to happen overnight. Taking a daily or weekly inventory can help regularly review your progress.

7. **Remind yourself of the benefits of recovery.** There are many benefits to recovery, even if it may not seem this way at a given time. This can help you during times when you think things are going too slowly or things aren't going well. This can help you see the "big picture" and the long-term benefits of recovery from co-occurring disorders.

8. **Make positive statements.** For example, let's say your son or daughter came home with a report card that wasn't as good as you had hoped. Rather than get critical, you might compliment them on their good grades and tell them you want to help them improve their other grades. Or, suppose a friend or someone whom you work with does something nice for you. Tell them you appreciate what they did. Show your gratitude.

9. **Write in a journal.** Write down positive thoughts or things that happen to you. Write at least a couple of positive statements each day or week.

10. **Read recovery literature.** Many good books on recovery can help you continue to learn ways to make positive changes in your thinking. Go to your local library or a bookstore, or search the Internet. Or, ask your therapist or doctor for other readings.

11. **Recite the slogans or the Serenity Prayer.** Slogans used in Twelve-Step programs such as "this too will pass," "think before you drink (or drug)" or "one day at a time" can help during rough times.

28. Spirituality

Spirituality refers to your sense of meaning in life and your connection to God, a Higher Power or others. It involves your values and the relationships and activities in your life that bring you meaning, purpose and direction. Spirituality encompasses your faith and religious practices. While you don't have to be associated with a "formal" religion to be spiritual, many people find it helpful to participate in a religion. Attending services and other religious practices can bring you comfort.

For some people, being of service to others is a way of showing spirituality. This may show in the work they do for a living or helping others by serving as a volunteer in a community program or organization (for example, at a nursing home, hospital, addiction treatment program, prison, as a "big brother" or "big sister"). In Twelve-Step recovery programs, there is much focus on spirituality and serving others by becoming a "sponsor." There are many ways you can be of service to others.

Recovery is a "we" process more than an "I" process. Therefore, becoming connected with and relying on other people and God or a Higher Power can aid your recovery. By sharing your recovery with others and working a "we" program, you not only "get" hope, strength, and support from others, you "give" it to others as well. Following are some questions to help focus on your spirituality.

1. What relationships, activities, or values give the most meaning and purpose to your life at this time? Explain your answer below.

    _____

    _____

    _____

    _____

    _____

2. Describe your own view of spirituality and what this means to you in recovery.

    _____

    _____

    _____

    _____

    _____

3. Describe ways in which you are or can be of service to other people.

    _____

    _____

    _____

    _____

4. Identify one area you would like to change or develop related to your spirituality. Then, state some steps you can take to work toward these changes.

_____

_____

_____

Strategies to Use Faith or Spirituality in Recovery

1. **Use your faith or religion.** This can give strength, guidance and add meaning to your life. Attend services, read spiritual literature or attend retreats to grow in spirituality. Talk with faith professionals.

2. **Rely on God or a Higher Power.** This can help you get through difficult times, give you peace or serenity and direction or meaning in life. You can also share gratitude to God for your blessings in your prayers or discussions with God or your Higher Power.

3. **Talk about spirituality.** Discuss spirituality issues in therapy, with a sponsor or at meetings. Share your ideas with others and hear their ideas.

4. **Use the Twelve Steps.** Many of the Twelve Steps, especially Steps 2, 3, 4, 5, 6, 7, 11, and 12 can help your spirituality.

5. **Focus on what has meaning in your life.** This may include your faith, relationships, activities and things important to you. Look at the world from the perspective of others, not just yourself.

6. **Give to others.** Be of service to others. Focus on the greater good of society. Think about what you can do to make the world a better place or help a specific person. Even small gestures can make a difference to others.

7. **Be positive.** Show love, compassion, kindness, gratitude, and forgiveness to others.

8. **Accept yourself.** Accept your limitations and be tolerant of your shortcomings or mistakes. You do not have to be perfect. Be kind to yourself when you make mistakes.

9. **Overcome negative emotions or feelings.** Work through guilt, shame, or other negative feelings with a therapist or sponsor. Managing emotions can reduce your risk of relapse to alcohol or drugs following a period of recovery.

SECTION VII

Lifestyle
Changes

29. My Daily Plan for Recovery

Recovery does happen one day at a time. Having a daily plan means taking steps to abstain from using alcohol or drugs and manage your other problems. It includes the "tools of recovery" that you use to make positive changes in yourself and your life. You need a "plan" to make sure you continue to focus on recovery.

Recovery Activity

1. Place a check mark next to recovery tools you use at least on a weekly basis:
   - ❑ AA, NA, CA meetings, or other addiction support group meetings.
   - ❑ DRA, other dual recovery or mental health support group meetings.
   - ❑ Discussions with a sponsor or friends in program (phone or face-to-face).
   - ❑ Working the Twelve Steps of AA/NA.
   - ❑ Individual or group therapy sessions; sessions with my psychiatrist.
   - ❑ Taking medications for a psychiatric disorder or addiction.
   - ❑ Praying, using a Higher Power or engaging in faith-based/religious services.
   - ❑ Reading recovery literature; writing in a journal or recovery workbook.
   - ❑ Talking self through cravings; practicing positive thinking.
   - ❑ Avoiding high risk people, places, things, having fun without using.
   - ❑ Other recovery tools (write in):

   _____

   _____

2. List benefits of regularly using your recovery tools.

   _____

   _____

   _____

3. List negative consequences of not using your recovery tools regularly.

   _____

   _____

   _____

   In early recovery, structure your time. The more active you are, and the less bored you are, the better your chances of staying sober. If you don't get involved in recovery activities or use recovery tools, you increase the chances of a relapse.

My Daily Schedule

	Sunday	Monday	Tuesday	Wednesday	Thursday	Friday	Saturday
6:00							
7:00							
8:00							
9:00							
10:00							
11:00							
12:00							
1:00							
2:00							
3:00							
4:00							
5:00							
6:00							
7:00							
8:00							
9:00							
10:00							
11:00							

30. Setting Goals

Goals give you direction and help focus your time and energy. Working hard at reaching your goals gives you a sense of satisfaction and accomplishment. On the other hand, without any goals in life, you are more likely to feel useless, bored, or depressed. And, your life is more likely to lack direction and structure which can raise the risk of relapse to alcohol or other drug use.

A goal refers to a process, a purpose, or some end that you wish to achieve. A goal can relate to learning information, developing new skills, or changing something about yourself, your relationships or lifestyle. Goals can be "general" or "specific." A *general goal* could be "to become a better parent." A *specific goal* could be "to get closer to your son by teaching him how to play a sport." Another general goal is "to become a better worker." A specific goal is "to learn how to use a computer so I am more efficient at work." "Losing weight and getting in shape" would be another general goal, whereas "losing 10 pounds by the end of summer" is a more specific goal.

Goals can be short-, medium-, or long-term. A *short-term goal* is something you want to achieve within three months, a *medium-term goal* is something you want to achieve in three to six months, and a *long-term goal* is something you want to achieve in six months or longer. Some goals are a one-shot deal, such as saving a specific amount of money for a down payment on a car, going on a vacation, completing a project or finishing a training program. Other goals are ongoing, especially goals related to changing yourself. For example, becoming more kind and loving or becoming a better spouse or parent is an ongoing goal that you continuously work toward. It is good to have a variety of goals. However, avoid setting too many goals or ones that are unreachable because you will feel bad if you don't achieve them.

Goals not only give you structure and a sense of purpose or direction, they can also become a yardstick against which you measure progress. For example, suppose you are lonely and isolated and set a goal of developing two new friendships within the next several months. If you actually develop these relationships, then you will know you have reached your goal.

Once you state your general or specific goal, then you need to figure steps you can take to reach your goal. These steps become your plan of action. Let's say, for example, that you set a general goal of "becoming closer to your family." You then have to figure how to go about getting closer to your family. You may accomplish this by regularly calling or visiting family members, inviting them to visit you, writing letters to them, sharing activities, or taking an interest in their lives.

Or, let's say you set a goal of "getting along better with my daughter." You may accomplish this by spending more time with her, taking an interest in her day-to-day activities, helping her with her homework or special projects, taking her to a movie or fun activity or telling her you love her. You may also work toward this goal by eliminating or reducing behaviors that interfere with your relationship such as snapping out angrily at her whenever she makes a mistake or belittling her if she doesn't do as well as you think she should in her school work.

You can develop goals in any area of your life. Following are examples:
1. **Your substance use disorder:** learning to stay off drugs or cope with desires to get high.
2. **Your psychiatric disorder:** learning to manage your symptoms.
3. **Your family:** getting closer to your parents by becoming more involved in their lives; improving your ability to resolve differences and conflicts with your spouse or becoming more affectionate.

4. **Your friendships and relationships:** expanding your social network or making new friends with whom you can share interests.
5. **Your interpersonal style:** learning to say no to others when you don't want to do things they ask of you or learning to express your ideas without worrying too much about what other people think.
6. **Your physical health:** improving your diet, losing weight, stopping smoking or getting in better physical shape.
7. **Your psychological or mental health:** expressing positive or negative feelings; changing negative thoughts or increasing the number of positive thoughts that you have each day; becoming less impulsive.
8. **Your spirituality:** developing a relationship with God or your Higher Power or becoming more active in religion.
9. **Your lifestyle:** learning a new hobby or sport or spending more time having fun; working toward a degree or toward finishing a training program; improving your job skills; budgeting your money or saving for the future.

After setting goals and developing an initial plan of action, share your ideas with your therapist, sponsor or a friend. Elicit their input and feedback on your goals and plan.

Review your goals regularly so you can assess your progress. If you aren't making progress, figure out if your goal is too high or unrealistic. Also, figure out if your plan needs changed or if there are other barriers to reaching your goals. It isn't unusual for goals and steps to achieve goals to be modified as time goes on.

Be sure to reward yourself, both for progress toward reaching your goals and for efforts you put forth. Even if you don't reach a particular goal, if you've done your best, then be happy with your efforts. Some goals are going to be harder to reach than others. Don't be afraid of failure, either. You can't grow as a person if you don't make mistakes.

Recovery Activity

(1) One *short-term goal* I want to achieve within the next three months is:

_____

_____

Steps I can take to reach this goal include:

_____

_____

_____

_____

(2) One *medium-term goal* I want to achieve within the next three to six months is:

_____

_____

Steps I can take to reach this goal include:

_____

_____

_____

_____

(3) One *long-term goal* I want to achieve within the next six to twelve months is:

_____

_____

Steps I can take to reach this goal include:

_____

_____

_____

_____

31. *Financial Issues in Recovery*

Addiction often causes financial problems as a result of money spent for alcohol or other drugs.[1] Addiction to expensive drugs or gambling often leads to big debts. Financial problems are also caused by missing work or losing a job. It is not uncommon to fall behind in paying bills or even go broke. Some end up losing everything they owned.

Your family may have experienced financial difficulties because of your addiction. Some families have trouble meeting their basic needs for medical or dental care, housing, food, clothing, education and recreation. A lack of consistent income, low income or poor money management can lead to anxiety and feelings of insecurity with your family.

Answer the following questions to help you plan for your financial recovery:

1. How much money would you estimate you spent on alcohol or other drugs during the: past month? _____ past year? _____

2. How much income in the past year would you estimate you lost due to missing work or losing jobs as a result of your problem? _____

3. How much of a drug debt or court/lawyer expense do you still have? _____

4. Describe other ways you or your family were affected financially by your addiction.

    _____

    _____

    _____

    _____

    _____

5. Describe steps you can take to begin getting your financial situation in order.

    _____

    _____

    _____

    _____

    _____

Financial issues can also be discussed with your counselor or AA/NA sponsor. Don't hesitate to seek the advice of a financial counselor if you think your situation warrants this. You may even wish to learn how to budget your money or manage a checking and/or savings account. (The next section will give you detailed information on handling money and debts.)

Some addicts associate having money with getting high. They feel they are more at risk to use if they have enough money for drugs. This attitude reflects denial and "stinking thinking." If you think like this, be sure to talk about it with your counselor and/or sponsor.

Strategies for Handling Money and Debt

1. **Keep track of your spending.** To get a handle on where your money goes, keep track of all your spending for a couple of months. This will help you more clearly see spending patterns. Tracking your spending can help you identify areas where you can cut down your spending. Using a budget book is an excellent way of tracking your spending and keeping a running account of how you spend your money.

2. **Develop and follow a written budget.** A budget helps you see the "big picture" in terms of how much you earn, how much you spend and what you spend your money on. Keeping a budget is a way to check your progress toward financial goals such as saving money or reducing debts. Following a budget can also help you prepare for expenses such as car insurance or holiday gifts. Review your budget at least monthly to help you see where your money is going, and to help you identify changes in spending habits that are needed. If you are on a limited income, live on public assistance or Supplemental Security Income (SSI), it is important to have a budget to make your income stretch.

3. **Live within your financial means.** If you spend more money than you bring in, then you are not living within your means. The longer you continue spending more money than you bring in, the deeper in debt you will go. Following a budget and developing a long-term financial plan are two ways of helping figure out ways to live within your means.

4. **Review your progress regularly.** Review your financial plan every week at first. This will help determine if you are reaching your goals or need to change your goals or methods. If your financial situation changes, your plan will have to be modified.

5. **Eliminate or reduce loans and charge cards.** Much money is wasted in interest paid on loans and charge cards. Charge cards may have interest rates almost as high as 30 percent. Loans may also have high interest rates. There are certain financial lenders whose interest rates are much higher than banks. Paying off loans and credit cards is one of the first steps to getting your financial house in order. Not only does this prevent money from being wasted in paying interest charges, but this also reduces the amount of money you have to pay out of your budget every month to meet the loan or credit card payments. While loans and credit card purchases are sometimes necessary, there are cases when they are not. If you are buying something with a credit card, ask yourself if you would buy this item if you had to pay cash. Ask yourself if you really need this item. Guard against impulsive buying with credit cards.

6. **Shop around for the best interest rates if you need a loan.** If you need a loan for a car, home improvement or for some other reason, check different lending institutions to compare interest rates. A difference of 1–2 percent on a car loan, for example, can mean saving $20 or more a month on your payment.

7. **Avoid loan sharks.** If you borrow from a loan shark, you will pay extremely high interest and this will throw you deeper into debt.

8. **Avoid aimless shopping and impulsive buying.** Don't shop when you don't need anything or you want to "look around." If you avoid aimless shopping you decrease the chances of impulsive buying. Most things bought on impulse are not things you "need," but things you "want."

9. **Think ahead to the future.** Regularly put aside money, even if only a small amount. The years fly by more quickly than you realize. Thinking ahead helps you plan for your future whether it

relates to buying a house or car, financing your child's education, or planning your retirement. Most employers offer retirement programs. If your employer's retirement program requires you to make a contribution from your paycheck, make sure you do this rather than take the money in your paycheck. This not only helps build for your future financial security, but reduces the amount of federal and state taxes taken from your pay. To protect your family, it is good to have life and disability insurance. If you are the sole support of your family, their security could be greatly jeopardized if you had a serious injury or illness and couldn't work, or if you died.

10. **Cut down expenses and increase savings.** There are a lot of "little" ways that you can cut down expenses and increase the money available for debt reduction or saving. You can buy food items and other household items in bulk quantity. Look for special sales or discount stores. If you are on a limited income and can't afford to buy in large quantities, get some friends to pitch in together to buy bulk quantities so you all can stretch your money. You can also save if you buy generic food and medicine products. Look for some things you need at yard sales, garage sales, estate sales, or advertised for sale by individuals in the newspaper. Other ways to reduce expenses include: taking your lunch to work, carpool to work, use the library instead of buying books, shop from a list and buy only items on your list, do not shop on an empty stomach, and rent or borrow items you seldom use instead of buying them.

11. **Use a financial counselor or consultant if needed.** If you are over your head in debt or over-whelmed with financial matters, discuss your situation with a financial counselor or consultant. This person can help you figure out your financial plan, whether it's simply to get control over your debts or to develop an investment plan for the future.

12. **Develop a financial plan (short- and long-term).** Money is no different than any other area of life in that if you develop goals and specific plans to follow to reach these goals, you are more likely to achieve them. A plan gives you a sense of direction. Your plan should include short- and long-term goals and should be in writing. If you are married or involved in a close relation-ship where money and assets are shared, this plan should be developed jointly with your spouse or partner so you both have input and agree on strategies. Working together is essential if a plan is to be developed in a way that considers both of your ideas and interests. It also gives you a greater chance that your plan will actually be followed.

32. The Importance of Follow-up after Rehab or Hospital-Based Treatment

If you received treatment in an inpatient or residential facility, you need to have a follow-up plan to continue your recovery. This plan addresses the problems you will work on once you are discharged. It outlines changes you want to make, resources you will use and steps you will take to reach your goals. Your family or others may be a source of support in putting together a follow-up plan. Your ongoing plan may involve continued professional treatment as well as participation in mutual support programs such as AA, NA, DRA, or others.

Other Inpatient Programs

Your treatment team may recommend further residential care following your current hospital or residential stay. Some people who finish treatment in an inpatient psychiatric or co-occurring disorders program or addiction rehab need a halfway house program or therapeutic community program to help them continue their recovery. Others may need a residential program that is designed for those with mental health disorders.

Partial or Intensive Outpatient Programs (Day Hospital)

A *partial hospital* (PH) or *intensive outpatient program* (IOP) offers treatment for several hours a day (three or more hours per day), 3–7 days per week. The purposes of these programs are to ease the transition between the hospital and community living or to offer an intensive program that may help prevent the need for care in a psychiatric hospital or addiction rehab or detox program. These programs offer recovery groups, therapy groups, individual and family sessions, medication and referral to other services (medical, housing, case management, etc.). Some programs offer on-site AA, NA or DRA meetings. These programs may be connected with a psychiatric treatment facility or an addiction treatment facility. Depending on the program you attend, the primary focus may be on your psychiatric disorder, your addiction, or both.

Some mental health systems offer *vocational rehabilitation programs* (VRPs). These aim to help you learn skills related to preparing for a job (e.g., resume writing, use of computer, job interviewing, social skills).

Outpatient Services

If your illness was severe enough to require an inpatient stay in a psychiatric or addiction treatment program, follow-up outpatient care is needed. Outpatient care (sometimes called "aftercare") helps you continue building on the gains you made in the hospital or rehab program. It also helps you deal with the problems and adjustments you face as you continue your recovery from co-occurring disorders.

There are different types of outpatient treatment. These include individual, group, and family therapy. You may receive outpatient care from a private professional such a psychiatrist, psychologist, or other mental health professional, a community based mental health center, an addiction clinic, or other type of agency.

For many people, symptoms of psychiatric illness and/or addiction come back. Involvement in outpatient care helps you spot the warning signs early and helps you either prevent a relapse, or get the help you need should a relapse occur. It is important to keep your outpatient appointments, even if you feel a lot better than before you went to the hospital. Stopping outpatient care too early can contribute to a relapse.

Medications

Many types of psychiatric illness require medications, even after the symptoms of your illness are under control. You need to see a psychiatrist or physician on a regular basis if you are on medication for a psychiatric illness. A common relapse warning sign is stopping medications without first talking it over with a counselor or doctor. If you feel you no longer need or want to take medications, talk with your counselor and doctor *before* you make a decision.

For acute episodes of psychiatric illness, it is often recommended that you stay on medications for 4–12 months after your symptoms improve. Make sure you talk with your doctor so you know how long to continue medicines after you improve.

If you have a recurrent type of psychiatric illness or a chronic form of illness, remain on your medications. If you stop, your symptoms are likely to get worse.

Medications are used to detoxify those addicted to alcohol, opioids, benzodiazepines or barbiturates, reduce cravings or desires for alcohol or drugs, block the effects of street drugs or as replacement drugs for those addicted to heroin or other opioids.[1–5] Some alcoholics use a medication called disulfiram (Antabuse). This drug stays in the system up to ten to fourteen days after the last dose is taken. If an alcoholic drinks while using this medication, he or she will get very sick. The idea is, if Antabuse is in one's system and there is a desire to drink, drinking may be put off until the Antabuse is out of the system. This essentially buys the alcoholic time and often within a few hours or days the desire to drink leaves. Naltrexone or vivitrol (ReVia) or acamprosate (Campral) are other medications used to reduce the craving for alcohol.

Opiate addicts use naltrexone (Trexan) to block the euphoric effects of opioid drugs. The idea is that if heroin or another opiate drug is used while taking naltrexone, the high won't be experienced. This in turn will discourage the addict from future episodes of opiate use. Methadone and buprenorphine are used to detoxify those addicted to opioids as well as used to help them maintain a drug-free status.

Any medication used for the treatment of addiction should be used with therapy or counseling and mutual support programs such as AA, NA, or DRA.

Mutual Support Programs

Many people have found mutual support programs for addiction (AA, NA, CA, Crystal Meth Anonymous), psychiatric illness (Emotions Anonymous, EHA, Recovery International) or dual disorder (Dual Recovery Anonymous) beneficial to their ongoing recovery. Mutual support programs are groups of people with similar problems or illnesses helping each other. They meet regularly to discuss their illnesses and problems, as well as steps they can take to overcome these. For example, many groups use a Twelve-Step recovery program which is a suggested way of viewing your problems and recovery from them.

There are different types of Twelve-Step meetings. Some are "speaker" meetings where a person talks about his illness and recovery. Other meetings are "discussion" where common problems or concerns are discussed. You can go to as many meetings as you need. Some people, for example, go every day. Others go once or twice a week.

Twelve-Step programs can provide you with a guide, often referred to as a *sponsor*. A sponsor is someone recovering from one or more illnesses who can "teach you the ropes" about the program. This is someone who will attend meetings with you, guide you through working the Twelve Steps, or talk with you by phone when you need a friendly voice.

You should get a list of programs available in your community before you leave the hospital or rehabilitation program. You may need to attend many meetings at different locations before you find one or more to attend on a regular basis. Those who get active in these programs and use the "tools" (meetings, sponsor, readings, Twelve Steps, events) do better than those who do not get active. [13]

Mutual support meetings are also available for your family. You may wish to speak with them about attending meetings such as Al-Anon, Nar-Anon or those sponsored by the National Alliance on Mental Illness (groups for families in which a member has a psychiatric illness).

Recovery Activity

1. What treatment program will you attend once you are discharged from an inpatient or residential program?_____

   Name & Phone Number of Program: _____

   Type of Program: _____

   Date of Appointment: _____

2. What is your plan for mutual support group programs (AA, NA, DRA, or others)? How many meetings will you attend each week?_____

   How soon will you get a sponsor if you don't have one?_____

   Will you work the Twelve Steps? _____

3. What other services will you use to aid your recovery or help with other problems (including involving your family)?

   _____

   _____

   _____

   _____

   _____

   _____

33. Relapse Warning Signs

Relapse is common with addiction and psychiatric illness.[1-4] There are many warning signs of relapse to both addiction and psychiatric illness you should learn about. These signs may show over a period of days, weeks or longer. Or, they can show up quickly. Being aware of relapse warning signs puts you in a position to take action so you don't use alcohol or drugs and you lessen your chances of a full-blown relapse of your psychiatric symptoms.

Relapse warning signs may show in changes in your attitude, mood, behavior and daily habits.[5-6] Sometimes, relapse warning signs show in existing symptoms worsening since some psychiatric symptoms may not totally go away.[7-8] For example, Leslie has learned that she can live with a certain degree of anxiety. However, when her anxiety level rises significantly for a few days and she starts to avoid going out of her house, she knows this is a relapse warning sign. Shawn can live with voices (hallucinations) as long as he believes that he can ignore them and his voices do not lead him to making decisions that can harm his health or make him feel tortured.

Warning signs may be obvious. For example, John knows he's headed back to drug use when he blows off NA meetings and calls guys he used to party with. Kelli knows she's likely to experience her mania again when she stops taking her lithium on her own without even discussing her condition with her therapist or doctor.

Warning signs can also be "sneaky" and not appear to relate to your co-occurring disorders. For example, before Anthony uses alcohol or drugs again, he begins to become dishonest in small ways by lying to friends or family. In time, his dishonesty shows in scamming and conning others. Soon, he's back to lying to doctors to get drugs. Before Amy uses cocaine, she is likely to seek out others who use even though she believes at the time her intention is to stay drug-free.

Although everyone has their own set of warning signs there are common ones that many people with co-occurring disorders experience before an episode of psychiatric illness or alcohol and drug use. Use the list that follows to learn about these warning signs and develop a plan for coping with them.

Recovery Activity

If you have been in treatment before for either or both of your disorders, try to figure which if any of the following warning signs may have been present before a relapse by placing a check mark next to the signs you experienced. If this is your first time in recovery, check the signs below that you think could represent relapse warning signs in the future.

Attitude and Thought Changes
- ❑ Losing interest in your treatment or recovery plan
- ❑ Thinking treatment or medications aren't needed anymore
- ❑ Not caring about yourself or what happens to your life
- ❑ Increase in negative thinking about the future or your treatment
- ❑ Racing and confusing thoughts
- ❑ Paranoid thoughts
- ❑ Thinking about hurting yourself or suicide
- ❑ Thinking about hurting someone else

- ❑ Thinking you can use "some" alcohol or drugs and stay in control
- ❑ Missing the action of partying, using alcohol and drugs, or being with a "fast crowd"
- ❑ Increase in obsessive thoughts
- ❑ Thinking about ways to take advantage of others or break the law

Mood or Emotional Changes: Feeling More

- ❑ Sad or depressed
- ❑ Energetic, excited, "keyed up," or on top of the world
- ❑ Anxious, nervous, or on edge
- ❑ Fearful and afraid
- ❑ Guilty and shameful
- ❑ Bored, restless, or "empty"
- ❑ Shifts in moods from depression to mania
- ❑ Lonely
- ❑ Angry and hurt

Behavior Changes

- ❑ Missing or stopping treatment sessions with your therapist or doctor
- ❑ Cutting down or stopping AA, NA, dual recovery, or mental support group meetings
- ❑ Cutting down or stopping medications without discussing this with therapist or doctor
- ❑ Cutting down or stopping regular contact with sponsor or other support group members
- ❑ Withdrawing from other people and keeping to yourself
- ❑ Arguing more with others
- ❑ Cutting down or stopping hobbies or enjoyable activities
- ❑ Putting yourself in situations where there is pressure to use alcohol or drugs
- ❑ Talking much slower or faster than usual, or in a way that is confusing to others
- ❑ Dressing in strange or bizarre ways
- ❑ Acting in strange or bizarre ways
- ❑ Hurting yourself (e.g., you cut or burn yourself)
- ❑ Hurting someone else
- ❑ Getting involved in illegal activities or breaking the law again

Health Habits or Daily Routine Changes

- ❑ Sleeping a lot more or less than usual, or trouble falling or staying asleep
- ❑ Big change in energy level (much higher or lower than usual)
- ❑ Big change in appetite or eating habits (increase or decrease)
- ❑ Cutting down or stopping regular exercise
- ❑ Change in personal hygiene habits
- ❑ Big change in your regular routines for the day or week

If there are any other relapse warning signs you've experienced before, write these below:

_____

_____

_____

_____

_____

_____

Recovery Activity

Review the list of warning signs you checked. In the spaces below, write down five possible warning signs of relapse for both your psychiatric illness and your addiction. Keep in mind some of these warning signs may be similar in both of your disorders.

Choose one psychiatric illness and one addiction relapse warning sign and list some steps you can take to help you cope with these warning signs. First, review the example of Gerald at the end of this section to see one example of how you can do this recovery task.

Psychiatric Warning Sign _____

_____

Three Coping Strategies:

(1) _____

(2) _____

(3) _____

Addiction Warning Sign _____

Three Coping Strategies:

(1) _____

(2) _____

(3) _____

Example: Gerald's Warning Signs and Coping Strategies

"My biggest warning sign is thinking that I don't need medications, treatment, or support groups once I've been feeling good for a couple of months. To cope with these thoughts in the future I will: (1) immediately talk over these thoughts with my doctor or therapist; (2) ask myself why am I really wanting to stop treatment to figure out what's really going on; (3) tell myself that I'm not going to make any decision to drop out of treatment for at least another month to buy myself more time; (4) discuss this feeling at the next meeting of the manic depression support group that I attend; (5) remind myself of how I do so much better when I stay on my medications and stay in treatment even during periods in which I am doing well. I have to remind myself that I have a chronic disease that can only be treated by staying on medication and staying in treatment."

34. Coping with Emergencies and Suicidal Thinking

Since many psychiatric illnesses are chronic or recurrent conditions, there is a chance your symptoms can worsen or return.[1] Addiction is also a chronic condition so it is also possible that you can relapse.[2] Working a good recovery plan helps you lessen the chances of relapse. It also helps you spot early signs of relapse so you can take action that hopefully will prevent a full-blown relapse.

Preparing yourself ahead of time puts you in a position to handle setbacks, problems, or actual relapses. Should symptoms of either or both of your illnesses return, it is better to take quick action instead of waiting for weeks or months because things can get worse. For example, when Sean's thoughts became more confused and disorganized and his hallucinations worsened, he immediately told his therapist and doctor. His medicine was readjusted and his treatment team gave him extra support which enabled him to cope with this return of symptoms without going to the hospital or drinking alcohol, which he commonly did in the past when his symptoms worsened. LaWanda, recovering from crack addiction and depression, missed her therapy sessions and cut down on NA meetings after being clean for ten months. She then drank some alcohol and decided she no longer needed medications. Fortunately, she told her sponsor who advised LaWanda to see her therapist immediately. With the help of her therapist and NA sponsor, LaWanda was able to get back on track again before using crack and then becoming depressed and suicidal.

You should seek help right away if your psychiatric symptoms return, if you have some persistent symptoms that worsen, or if you use alcohol or drugs again. Many times, early action can prevent a full-blown relapse and prevent you from having to go to the hospital for detoxification or stabilization of severe psychiatric symptoms.

One of the reasons that it is good to develop an emergency plan ahead of time is that symptoms of your illness can impair your judgment and lead you to deny or minimize your relapse. Therefore, you should discuss your emergency plan with your treatment team, sponsor and family so others can help you should an emergency occur.

Suicidal Thinking

Suicidal thinking and behaviors represent one serious type of emergency.[3] Suicide is the eighth leading cause of death in the United States. Between 5 and 15 percent of adults have suicidal thoughts at some point in their lives. However, not everyone who thinks about suicide makes a plan, acts on suicidal thoughts, or follows their suicidal plan. Most people who make an attempt will not make a second one. However, some people make multiple attempts over time—these people are at the highest risk to complete suicide.

Suicidal thoughts and behaviors are higher among those with a mental disorder, addiction, or both. Major depression, bipolar illness, schizophrenia, and alcoholism are examples of specific disorders in which suicidal risk is high.

Women make more suicidal attempts than men, but men succeed more often because they use more lethal ways (e.g., weapons, hanging, poison). Suicidal attempts are also higher among the younger than older population, those with lower levels of education, the unemployed, whites, and those who are widowed, divorced, or single.

Recovery Activity

Answer the following questions to put together an emergency plan and review this with your counselor, spouse, and anyone else you think can help you.

1. Steps I can take if I use *any* alcohol or drugs are:

    _____

    _____

    _____

    _____

2. Steps I can take if I get *physically or mentally hooked* again are:

    _____

    _____

    _____

    _____

3. Steps I can take if my psychiatric symptoms worsen or return include:

    _____

    _____

    _____

    _____

4. I would need to go in to the hospital for help if I experienced these symptoms or behaviors:

    _____

    _____

    _____

    _____

5. My family, sponsor, or members of my recovery network can help me if I experience an emergency by taking the following steps:

    _____

    _____

    _____

    _____

Discuss your plan with people in your recovery network while you are doing well. Ask for help from your therapist or doctor in developing this plan.

Strategies to Manage Emergencies and Reduce Suicidal Risk

1. **Stay active in treatment and recovery.** Talk about your problems, suicidal thoughts, feelings or plans, relapses, or personal struggles with your counselor and/or doctor. Make sure that you keep all of your counseling and doctor's appointments so you get the most out of professional care. Stay connected to others in recovery by attending mutual support groups. Since emergencies do occur, active involvement in treatment and mutual support groups can help you nip these in the bud. Others can give you help and support during difficult times.

2. **Manage your emotions.** Sections 16–20 of this workbook provide specific ideas on managing different emotions, many of which are common among addiction and psychiatric disorders. Controlling and regulating your emotions can improve your mental health, reduce suicidal feelings, and improve the quality of your life.

3. **Use the support and help of others.** Sections 21–24 of this workbook provide ideas on building relationships and support. Recovery is not something you should do alone. Ask for help and support from others if you experience any type of emergency including: a recurrence of your psychiatric illness after a period of remission; a relapse to alcohol or drug use after a period of sobriety; a return or increase in suicidal thoughts and feelings; or other type of serious problem. By getting support and help from others, you can manage an emergency and lower your risk of relapse or suicide.

4. **Be alert for the warning signs of psychiatric or addiction relapse.** Knowing the signs of relapse puts you in a position to "catch" these early and take action. Warning signs can be obvious, or they may be subtle. Section 33 of this workbook lists some of the common warning signs associated with relapse of both types of disorders. Use this information to identify and manage relapse signs.

5. **Be alert for the warning signs of suicide.** Warning signs of suicide are often related to symptoms of a mental disorder such as depression, bipolar illness, or schizophrenia.[4] Warning signs include increased thoughts about suicide or that life isn't worth living; talking more about suicide; preparing for death by making out a will; giving away important possessions; feeling much more depressed or hopeless; significant decrease in interest in life; depressive symptoms (e.g., changes in your appetite, sleep, or energy); or increasing your alcohol or other drug use.

If you have previously attempted suicide or feel your risk is high, develop a written "safety" plan with the help of others. This safety plan can include the names and phone numbers of an emergency room, professionals you can call in time of crisis, friends or relatives you can call in times of crisis, and steps you can take to stay in control of your behaviors. Include your current diagnoses, psychiatric medications, and insurance information so this can be shared with others should there be a need for hospitalization.

References

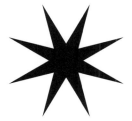

Chapter 2

1. L. N. Robins & D. A. Regier, eds., *Psychiatric Disorders in America: The Epidemiologic Catchment Area Study.* (New York, New York: The Free Press, 1991).

2. R. C. Kessler, K. A. McGonagle, & S. Zhao, "Lifetime and 12-month Prevalence of DSM-III-R Psychiatric Disorders in the United States: Results from the National Comorbidity Survey," *Archives of General Psychiatry.* 51 (1994): 8–19.

3. U.S. Department of Health and Human Services, *Substance Abuse Treatment for Persons with Co-Occurring Disorders,* DHHS Publication No. (SMA) 05-3992, (Rockville, Maryland: SAMHSA, 2005).

4. D. C. Daley & H. Moss, *Co-Occurring Disorders: Counseling Clients with Chemical Dependency and Mental Illness*, 3rd ed. (Center City, Minnesota: Hazelden, 2002).

5. D. C. Daley, I. M. Salloum, H. B. Moss, D. FitzGerald, & L. Kirisci, "Aftercare Treatment Entry and Adherence Rates among Discharged Psychiatric Inpatients with and without Substance Abuse Comorbidity" (unpublished data).

6. *Diagnostic and Statistical Manual of Mental Disorders (DSM-IV-TR)*, 4th ed. (Washington, D.C.: American Psychiatric Press, APA, 2000), 192–198.

7. Ibid., 198–199.

8. D. C. Daley & A. Douaihy, *Addiction and Mood Disorders.* (*New York, New York:* Oxford University Press, 2006).

9. D. C. Daley & A. Douaihy, *Depression Recovery Workbook.* (Apollo, Pennsylvania: Daley Publications, 2009).

10. F. K. Goodwin & K. R. Jamison, *Manic-Depressive Illness: Bipolar Disorders and Recurrent Depression*, 2nd ed. (New York, New York: Oxford University Press, 2007).

11. D. J. Stein, D. J. Kupfer & A. F. Schatzberg, eds. *Textbook of Mood Disorders.* (Washington, D.C.: American Psychiatric Publishing, Inc., 2006).

12. D. C. Daley. *Understanding Suicide and Addiction.* (Center City, Minnesota: Hazelden, 2003).

13. *Diagnostic and Statistical Manual of Mental Disorders (DSM-IV-TR)*, 4th ed. (Washington, D.C.: American Psychiatric Press, APA, 2000), 345–428.

14. Goodwin and Jamison, op. cit.

15. D. J. Stein, E. Hollander & B. O. Rothbaum, eds. *Textbook of Anxiety Disorders,* 2nd ed. (Washington, D.C.: American Psychiatric Publishing, Inc., 2010).

16. D. C. Daley & A. Douaihy, *Recovery from Anxiety Disorders.* (Apollo, Pennsylvania: Daley Publications, 2008).

17. *Diagnostic and Statistical Manual of Mental Disorders (DSM-IV-TR)*, 4th ed. (Washington, D.C.: American Psychiatric Press, APA, 2000), 443–456.

18. Ibid., 433–441.

19. Ibid., 456–463.

20. Ibid., 472–476.

21. Ibid., 463–468.

22. L. M. Najavits, *Seeking Safety: A Treatment Manual for PTSD and Substance Abuse.* (New York, New York: Guilford Press, 2002).

23. *Diagnostic and Statistical Manual of Mental Disorders (DSM-IV-TR)*, 4th ed. (Washington, D.C.: American Psychiatric Press, APA, 2000), 297–343.

24. J. A. Lieberman, T. S. Stroup & D. O. Perkins, eds. *Textbook of Schizophrenia.* (Washington, D.C.: American Psychiatric Publishing, Inc., 2006).

25. *Diagnostic and Statistical Manual of Mental Disorders (DSM-IV-TR)*, 4th ed. (Washington, D.C.: American Psychiatric Press, APA, 2000), 685–729.

26. J. M. Oldham, A. E. Skodol & D. S. Bender, eds., *Textbook of Personality Disorders.* (Washington, D.C.: American Psychiatric Publishing, Inc., 2005).

27. *Diagnostic and Statistical Manual of Mental Disorders (DSM-IV-TR)*, 4th ed. (Washington, D.C.: American Psychiatric Press, APA, 2000), 85–93.

28. R. A. Barkley, K. R. Murphy & M. Fischer, *ADHD in Adults: What the Science Says.* (New York, New York: Guilford Press, 2008).

29. D. C. Daley & M. E. Thase, *Dual Disorders Recovery Counseling,* 3rd ed. (Independence, Missouri: Independence Press, 2003).

30. F. K. Goodwin & K. R. Jamison, *Manic-Depressive Illness: Bipolar Disorders and Recurrent Depression,* 2nd ed. (New York, New York: Oxford University Press, 2007).

31. C. R. Cloninger, "Genetics of Addiction," in M. Galanter and H. D. Kleber, eds., *Textbook of Substance Abuse Treatment*, 3rd ed. (Washington, D.C.: American Psychiatric Publishing 2008), 17–28.

32. N. C. Andreasen, *Brave New Brain: Conquering Mental Illness in the Era of the Genome* (New York, New York: Oxford University Press, 2001).

33. National Institute on Drug Abuse, *Drugs, Brains, and Behavior: The Science of Addiction.* (Rockville, Maryland: NIDA, NIH Publication No. 08-5605, 2007).

34. D. C. Daley & G. A. Marlatt, *Overcoming Your Alcohol or Drug Problem: Effective Recovery Strategies.* Therapist Guide, 2nd ed. (New York, New York: Oxford University Press, 2006).

35. National Institute on Drug Abuse, *Drugs, Brains, and Behavior: The Science of Addiction.* (Rockville, Maryland: NIDA, NIH Publication No. 08-5605, 2007).

36. R. E. Drake, K. T. Mueser, R. E. Clark, & M. A. Wallach, "The Course, Treatment, and Outcome of Substance Disorder in Persons with Severe Mental Illness," *American Journal of Orthopsychiatry* 66, no. 1 (1996): 41–51.

37. D. C. Daley & H. Moss, *Co-Occurring Disorders: Counseling Clients with Chemical Dependency and Mental Illness*, 3rd ed. (Center City, Minnesota: Hazelden, 2002).

Chapter 3

1. K. Minkoff & C. Ajilore, *Co-Occurring Psychiatric and Substance Disorders in Managed Care Systems: Standards of Care, Practice Guidelines, Workforce Competencies, and Training Curricula,* Report of the Center for Mental Health Services Managed Care Initiative (Philadephia, Pennsylvania: published by the authors, 1998).

2. K. Minkoff & R. E. Drake, *Dual Diagnosis of Major Mental Illness and Substance Disorder.* (San Francisco, California: Jossey-Bass, 1991).

3. J. Horsfall, M. Cleary, G. E. Hunt & G. Walter "Psychosocial treatments for people with co-occurring severe mental illness and substance use disorders (dual diagnosis): a review of empirical evidence," *Harvard Review of Psychiatry*, 17, no. 3 (2009): 24–34.

4. R. E. Drake, E. L. O'Neal & M. A. Wallach, "A systematic review of psychosocial research on psychosocial interventions for people with co-occurring severe mental and substance use disorders," *Journal of Substance Abuse Treatment*, 34 (2008): 123–138.

5. D. C. Daley & A. Douaihy, *Recovery and Relapse Prevention for Co-Occurring Disorders.* (Apollo, Pennsylvania: Daley Publications, 2010).

6. D. C. Daley, I. M. Salloum, & A. Jones-Barlock, "Integrating a Co-Occurring Disorders Program in an Acute-Care Psychiatric Hospital," *Psychosocial Rehabilitation Journal* 15, no. 2 (1991): 45–56.

7. D. C. Daley & M. E. Thase, *Co-Occurring Disorders Recovery Counseling: Integrated Treatment for Substance Use and Mental Health Disorders,* 3rd ed. (Independence, Missouri: Independence Press, 2003).

8. D. C. Daley & A. Zuckoff, *Improving Treatment Compliance: Counseling and Systems Strategies for Substance Use and Co-Occurring Disorders.* (Center City, Minnesota: Hazelden, 1999).

9. A. T. McLellan, D. C. Lewis, C. P. O'Brien, & H. D. Kleber, "Drug Dependence, a Chronic Medical Illness: Implications for Treatment, Insurance, and Outcomes Evaluation," *Journal of the American Medical Association.* 284, no. 13 (2000): 1689–1695.

10. National Institute on Alcohol Abuse and Alcoholism, *Alcohol and Health: Tenth Special Report to the U. S. Congress.* (Rockville, Maryland: NIAAA, 2000).

11. National Institute on Drug Abuse, *Principles of Drug Addiction Treatment: A Research-Based Guide.* (Rockville, Maryland: NIDA, 2009).

12. D. C. Daley & H. Moss, *Co-Occurring Disorders: Counseling Clients with Chemical Dependency and Mental Illness*, 3rd ed. (Center City, Minnesota: Hazelden, 2002).

Chapter 9

1. J. O. Prochaska, J. C. Norcross, & C. C. DiClemente, *Changing for Good.* (New York, New York: William Morrow and Company, 1994).

2. M. E. Thase, "Relapse and Recurrence in Unipolar Major Depression: Short-term and Long-term Approaches," *Journal of Clinical Psychiatry* 51, No. 6 (1990): 51–57.

3. D. C. Daley & M. E. Thase, *Co-Occurring Disorders Recovery Counseling: Integrated Treatment for Substance Use and Mental Health Disorders*, rev. ed. (Independence, Missouri: Herald House/Independence Press, 2000).

4. Prochaska, Norcross & DiClemente, op. cit.

Chapter 13

1. D. C. Daley & M. E. Thase, *Co-Occurring Disorders Recovery Counseling: Integrated Treatment for Substance Use and Mental Health Disorders*, 3rd ed. (Independence, Missouri: Herald House/Independence Press, 2003).

2. M. M. Lineham, *Skills Training Manual for Treating Borderline Personality Disorder.* (New York, New York: Guilford Press, 1993).

3. D. C. Daley & G. A. Marlatt, *Overcoming Your Alcohol or Drug Problem: Client Workbook.* (New York, New York: Oxford University Press, 2006), 41–52.

Chapter 14

1. D. C. Daley & A. Douaihy, *Recovery and Relapse Prevention for Co-Occurring Disorders.* (Apollo, Pennsylvania: Daley Publications, 2010).

2. D. C. Daley & M. E. Thase, *Co-Occurring Disorders Recovery Counseling: Integrated Treatment for Substance Use and Mental Health Disorders*, 3rd ed. (Independence, Missouri: Herald House/Independence Press, 2003).

Chapter 15

1. D. C. Daley & G. A. Marlatt, *Overcoming Your Alcohol or Drug Problem: Client Workbook.* (New York, New York: Oxford University Press, 2006), 59–68.

Chapter 16

1. D. C. Daley, *Managing Anger Workbook*, 3rd ed. (Apollo, Pennsylvania: Daley Publications, 2004).
2. M. Salloum, M. E. Thase & D. C. Daley, *Male Depression, Alcoholism, and Violence.* (London, England: Martin Dunitz Publishers, 2000).
3. Mills, J. F., Kroner, D. G., & Morgan, R. D. *Clinician's Guide to Violence Risk Assessment.* (New York, New York: Guilford Press, 2011).

Chapter 17

1. D. C. Daley & I. M. Salloum, *Understanding Anxiety Disorders and Addiction Workbook*, 2nd ed. (Center City, Minnesota: Hazelden, 2003).
2. D. C. Daley & A. Douaihy, *Anxiety Disorders Recovery Workbook.* (Apollo, Pennsylvania: Daley Publications, 2008).

Chapter 19

1. D. C. Daley & M. E. Thase, *Understanding Depression and Addiction Workbook*, 2nd ed. (Center City, Minnesota: Hazelden, 2003).
2. D. C. Daley & A. Douaihy, *Addiction and Mood Disorders.* (New York, New York: Oxford University Press, 2006).
3. D. J. Kupfer, E. Frank, J. Perel et al., "Five-year Outcome for Maintenance Therapies in Recurrent Depression," *Journal of General Psychiatry* 49 (1993): 769–773.

Chapter 20

1. D. C. Daley & A. Douaihy, *Managing Emotions.* (Apollo, Pennsylvania: Daley Publications, 2004).
2. D. C. Daley & A. Douaihy, *Gratitude Workbook.* (Apollo, Pennsylvania: Daley Publications, 2010).

Chapter 21

1. D. C. Daley & J. S. Spear, *A Family Guide to Coping with Co-Occurring Disorders: Addiction and Psychiatric Illness*, 3rd ed. (Center City, Minnesota: Hazelden, 2003).
2. D. C. Daley & A. Douaihy, *A Family Guide to Addiction and Recovery.* (Apollo, Pennsylvania: Daley Publications, 2010).
3. K. T. Mueser, S. M. Glynn, C. Cather et al., "Family Intervention for Co-Occurring Substance Use and Severe Psychiatric Disorders," *Addictive Behaviors.* 34 (2009): 867–877.

Chapter 22

1. D. C. Daley & G. A. Marlatt, *Overcoming Your Alcohol or Drug Problem, Client Workbook* (New York, New York: Oxford University Press, 2006), 83–88.
2. G. A. Marlatt & D. Donovan, *Relapse Prevention.* 2nd ed. (New York, New York: Guilford Press, 2005).

Chapter 23

1. D. C. Daley & G. A. Marlatt, *Overcoming Your Alcohol or Drug Problem, Client Workbook.* (New York, New York: Oxford University Press, 2006), 99–104.
2. D. C. Daley & A. Douaihy, *Sober Relationships and Support System in Recovery: For Substance use or Co-Occurring Disorders,* 2nd ed. (Apollo, Pennsylvania: Daley Publications, 2010).

Chapter 24

1. D. C. Daley, D. Donovan & A. Douaihy, *Using Twelve-Step Programs in Recovery*, 2nd ed. (Apollo, Pennsylvania: Daley Publications, 2010).
2. Many of the mutual support programs for substance use disorders, other addictions, psychiatric illness, and co-occurring disorders publish recovery literature that describes their programs and how to benefit from them.

Chapter 26

1. R. Weiss & D. C. Daley, *Understanding Personality Problems and Addiction Workbook*, 2nd ed. (Center City, Minnesota: Hazelden, 2003).

Chapter 27

1. Many books have been written about beliefs and thinking, and their impact on disorders. These books also give advice on strategies to change thinking, which can have a positive impact on mood and behavior.
2. D. C. Daley & G. A. Marlatt, *Overcoming Your Alcohol or Drug Problem, Client Workbook.* (New York, New York: Oxford University Press, 2006), 69–74.
3. D. C. Daley, *Overcoming Negative Thinking.* (Center City, Minnesota: Hazelden, 1991).

Chapter 31

1. D. C. Daley, *Money and Recovery Workbook.* (Apollo, Pennsylvania: Daley Publications, 2005).

Chapter 32

1. A. J. Saxon, ed., "Pharmacologic Interventions" in R. K. Ries, D. A. Fiellin, S. C. Miller & R. Saitz, eds., *Principles of Addiction Medicine,* 4th ed. (New York, New York: Lippincott Williams & Wilkins, 2009), 629–743.
2. D. C. Daley, A. Douaihy & A. Hahn, *Detox Recovery Workbook.* (Apollo, Pennsylvania: Daley Publication, 2010).
3. D. C. Daley & G. A. Marlatt, *Overcoming Your Alcohol or Drug Problem, Client Workbook.* (New York, New York: Oxford University Press, 2006), 113–124.
4. I. M. Salloum, M. E. Thase, & D. C. Daley, *Male Depression, Alcoholism and Violence.* (London, England: Martin Dunitz Publishers, 2000).
5. J. R. Volpicelli, A. I. Alterman, M. Hayashida, & C. P. O'Brien, "Naltrexone in the Treatment of Alcohol Dependence," *Archives of General Psychiatry.* 49, no. 11 (1992): 876–880.

Chapter 33

1. A. Douaihy, D. C. Daley, G. A. Marlatt & C. R. Spotts, "Relapse Prevention: Clinical Models and Intervention Strategies," in R. K. Ries, D. A. Fiellin, S. C. Miller & R. Saitz, eds., *Principles of Addiction Medicine,* 4th ed. (New York, New York: Lippincott Williams & Wilkins, 2009), 883–898.
2. G. A. Marlatt & D. Donovan, *Relapse Prevention,* 2nd ed. (New York, New York: Guilford Press, 2004).
3. D. C. Daley & A. Douaihy, *Recovery and Relapse Prevention for Co-Occurring Disorders.* (Apollo, Pennsylvania: Daley Publications, 2010).
4. M. E. Thase, "Relapse and Recurrence in Unipolar Major Depression: Short-term and Long-term Approaches," *Journal of Clinical Psychiatry* 51, no. 6 (1990): 51–57.
5. D. C. Daley, *Relapse Prevention Workbook: For Recovering Alcoholics and Drug Dependent Persons*, 5th ed. (Apollo, Pennsylvania: Daley Publications, 2009).
6. T. T. Gorski & M. Miller, *Counseling for Relapse Prevention.* (Independence, Missouri: Herald House/Independence Press, 1982).
7. D. C. Daley, *Preventing Relapse*, 2nd ed. (Center City, Minnesota: Hazelden, 2003).
8. D. C. Daley & L. Roth, *When Symptoms Return: A Guide to Relapse in Psychiatric Illness*, 2nd ed. (Holmes Beach, Florida: Learning Publications, 2001).

Chapter 34

1. D. C. Daley & L. Roth, *When Symptoms Return: A Guide to Relapse in Psychiatric Illness*, 2nd ed. (Holmes Beach, Florida: Learning Publications, 2001).
2. D. C. Daley, *Relapse Prevention Workbook: For Recovering Alcoholics and Drug Dependent Persons*, 5th ed. (Apollo, Pennsylvania: Daley Publications, 2009).
3. D. C. Daley, *Understanding Suicide and Addiction.* (Center City, Minnesota: Hazelden, 2003).

Helpful
Resources

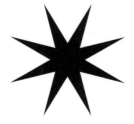

There are many resources on addiction, relapse, relapse prevention, and recovery. These include informational resources (books, guides, workbooks, and electronic media) as well as self-help programs. In addition to the list which follows, resources can be accessed on the Internet through bookstores, publishers of recovery literature or by conducting a search of key terms or words such as: addiction, alcohol abuse, alcohol addiction, alcohol dependence, or alcoholism, drug abuse, drug addiction or drug dependency, families and addiction, recovery from addiction, relapse, relapse prevention, or the name of a specific substance, person, or organization associated with treatment of addiction or recovery.

Alcoholics Anonymous	*www.aa.org*
Al-Anon Family Groups	*www.al-anon.org*
Dennis C. Daley, Ph.D.	*www.drdenniscdaley.com*
Dual Recovery Anonymous (DRA)	*www.draonline.org*
Harvard Health Publications	*www.health.harvard.edu*
Hazelden Educational Materials	*www.hazelden.org*
Herald House/Independence Press	*www.heraldhouse.org*
Narcotics Anonymous	*www.na.org*
Nar-Anon Family Groups	*www.nar-anon.org*
National Institute of Mental Health	*www.nimh.nih.org*
National Institute on Alcohol Abuse and Alcoholism	*www.niaaa.nih.gov*
National Institute on Drug Abuse	*www.nida.nih.gov*
Substance Abuse and Mental Health Services Administration	*www.samhsa.gov*

Notes

Notes